MAYBE
IT'S YOUR
MEDICATIONS

MAYBE IT'S YOUR MEDICATIONS

HOW TO AVOID UNNECESSARY DRUG THERAPY AND ADVERSE DRUG REACTIONS

DR. HEDVA BARENHOLTZ LEVY, PHARMD

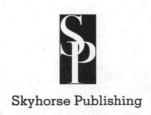

Skyhorse Publishing

Skyhorse Publishing books may be purchased in bulk at special discounts for sales promotion, corporate gifts, fund-raising, or educational purposes. Special editions can also be created to specifications. For details, contact the Special Sales Department, Skyhorse Publishing, 307 West 36th Street, 11th Floor, New York, NY 10018 or info@skyhorsepublishing.com.

Skyhorse® and Skyhorse Publishing® are registered trademarks of Skyhorse Publishing, Inc.®, a Delaware corporation.

Visit our website at www.skyhorsepublishing.com.

10 9 8 7 6 5 4 3 2 1

Library of Congress Cataloging-in-Publication Data is available on file.

Cover design by Kai Texel
Cover image: Getty Images

Print ISBN: 978-1-5107-7483-4
Ebook ISBN: 978-1-5107-7484-1

Printed in the United States of America

Contents

Part V: Strategies for Safer Medication Use

List of Tables and Figures

Chapter 17

Chapter 19

To my husband, Don, for your unending support.
To my mother and father always.

Introduction

"I think I'm taking too many pills, but my doctor says I need them all."

"Is it okay for me to take all of these medications together—and with these supplements, too?"

"My mom's behavior just isn't the same."

Maybe you can relate to these concerns, being a bit wary about taking medications. Or perhaps you don't worry too much about your medications.

"I only take what the doctor prescribes."

"My doctors all look at my medications."

"I get my medications every month at the pharmacy."

Are the medications we take helpful or harmful? Medications have a very important role in keeping us healthy and extending our lives; there is no doubt. But when do we cross the line from taking the right number and mix of drugs to keep us healthy to taking more than are necessary? All too often an unrecognized adverse drug reaction is mistaken for a new medical condition, or worse: a symptom of getting older. But who stops to question the medications?

This book is about safe medication use. It focuses on older adults as defined in the medical field as anyone age sixty-five and older, but the principles apply to people of any age who take medications. Older adults make up the fastest growing segment of our population. They have more long-term health conditions and take more medication than any other age group, and medication use is associated with far more problems in older individuals compared to younger adults.

Our society has become reliant on medications to fix our problems. We are inundated with messages of the benefits of drugs, from advertisements for prescription drugs to over-the-counter products and dietary supplements. We are left with a medication-use problem in America that is marked by extensive prescribing. And we have a health system where older adults take a growing list of medications and then fall through the cracks, with those medications often continued for life and never scrutinized.

As we strive to age independently and stay as healthy as possible, inappropriate use of medications can get in the way. Healthy aging requires that we are respectful of how medications can help us manage our health, but also recognize the limitations of these medications. In general, commercial messaging about medications tends to overemphasize the positive, and as a society, we are conditioned that a pill is the answer. Yet plenty of medications offer only small or questionable benefits. In some cases, the benefits in older adults can be outweighed by potential adverse effects. Problems that can occur when older adults take more and more medications are wide ranging and can ultimately negatively affect one's quality of life. We need to put the brakes on over-prescribing and find a path to more careful and intentional use of medications. While medical training and health systems are beginning to address the problem of excessive medication use, individual patients and consumers can take action now to make a difference in their own health care.

My goal in writing this book is to stop the cascade of medication overuse and misuse. We need to begin talking about our medications to better understand which ones are of benefit and which ones might no longer be needed or possibly are harmful. I want to empower individuals of any age—but especially older adults—to become educated consumers and wiser medication users. *Maybe It's Your Medications* provides information about the scope of medication-related problems, why these problems matter, and what individuals can do to reduce the risk of experiencing a serious problem.

I have been a geriatric specialist pharmacist for over twenty-five years, working with older adults and their adult children to provide personalized medication evaluations. My focus is on identifying and addressing medication-related problems, educating individuals and family members about their medications, and communicating with physicians to optimize patients' drug therapy. Through the years, I have accumulated far too many examples of errors that occur in how we prescribe, monitor, dispense, and take medications—errors that could have been prevented. Many of these stories are sprinkled throughout the chapters that follow to help give you a sense of the vast ways in which medication use can go awry, despite the best of intentions. We need informed patients and consumers to be more engaged in their health care, and especially medication use, to prevent errors and other problems associated with medication use.

If I dwell on the negative side of medications, it is because it needs to be talked about. We need to have a greater appreciation of the range of problems that can occur with medications—including both prescription and nonprescription drugs. Today's drug therapy options have the potential to be extremely effective, but those benefits come with a greater potential for harm if the drugs are not used properly. Couple this with a prescribing epidemic, an aging population, and a healthcare workforce that is not sufficiently trained in the care of older adults (geriatrics), and we are in the midst of a setup for a medication crisis in the United States. This book is a wake-up call for everyone who takes medications and for healthcare professionals who care for older adults.

Importantly, this book is NOT many things. It is not a replacement for your pharmacists or physicians. It is not a manual of good and bad drugs. It certainly is not a source of detailed information about specific drugs. The drug names I include in these pages are merely examples or part of a patient's story. Other drug information resources exist, and if you have a question about a drug that I mention here, please take it to your pharmacist, physician, or another trusted professional.

This book is not a permission slip to make changes in your drug therapy without first talking to your physicians and pharmacists. You cannot know everything about medications, and I do not expect you to have the knowledge of a pharmacist. However, you are able to understand the basis for why we need to care about medication use in older adults. And you can learn how to advocate for yourselves and your loved ones regarding medication-related questions.

On the other hand, this book IS a resource on how to think about medications in a different way. It explains why pharmacy issues are unique for older patients. It is a guidebook for older adults and anyone who works with older adults to use medications more safely and effectively. It is an educational tool for everyone who is interested in preventing medication-related problems in older adults.

Our society is aging, and medication issues will continue to loom large. This makes it imperative for everyone, including healthcare professionals, to pay more attention to how we can work together to reduce the preventable costs associated with medication-related problems. Start unraveling your questions about medications and your concerns about the possible harm they might cause. Yes, medications can cause problems, but if you know why many problems happen and what you can do to prevent them, you have won a major battle. It takes everyone on the healthcare team to reduce risks associated with medication use. And you are on that team. You can learn to play in the game. This book contains advice, information, and strategies on where and how to begin. Begin by understanding what each of your medications is for and how you can avoid taking unnecessary drugs or drugs that may be of limited benefit. If you want to master your medication list, read on. Maybe it's your medications, and maybe it's not, but we need to talk about it.

Part I

Medication Use in an Aging Population

Chapter 1

The Growing Medication-Use Problem

We have a perfect storm arriving that is causing a new kind of medication problem in the United States. An aging population, escalating medication use and drug costs, and improper or inappropriate use of medications have led to a heavy burden both on individuals and on strained health care systems. It is time to do something about it.

More than ever, we rely on medications for our well-being, especially as we get older and acquire new diagnoses. Medications are a key pillar in managing chronic health conditions, and millions of Americans take them to live longer, healthier lives. On the other hand, medications have become a crutch to us. They are widely available both with and without a prescription, and commercial advertisements bombard us with their benefits. Risks commonly are presented in small print or spoken quickly and compete with positive imagery. For most people, it is second nature to seek medications to treat minor ailments, mask discomfort, or provide quick relief. Maybe the body would heal on its own or with treatments that do not involve a drug, but we rarely give that a chance. Too many individuals are happy to take a pill rather than do the heavier lift of looking at their lifestyle choices. While undoubtedly medications are irreplaceable in certain situations, overuse and misuse of drug therapy has its consequences.

In my experience as a pharmacist meeting with patients about their drug therapy, many individuals do not know about their medicines—what they are treating and what the goals of therapy are. A common conversation goes something like this one that I had with George, seventy-two years old and living on his own. As I sat with him at his kitchen table and asked him about each of his medications, I came to his prescription bottle for omeprazole. I asked him if he knew why he took it. He said he did not; only that "his doctor prescribed it for [him]."

"It's a stomach medicine," I offered, hoping to jog his memory. I explained that it decreases stomach acid. Maybe he had been diagnosed with a stomach ulcer, bleeding in the stomach, or severe indigestion, I suggested, hoping to uncover a valid clinical reason for it.

"No," George paused. "But last winter, I told my doctor that I had a pain in my stomach, and I think maybe that's when he gave me the pill." I next asked him how the stomach pain was doing, after taking the drug for roughly eight months. Improvement should have been evident within two weeks and the problem resolved by eight weeks for most acid-related diagnoses for which omeprazole commonly is prescribed. He told me the pain was no different. "Still there," he said.

This scenario likely sounds a little familiar to you. George did not know why the medication was prescribed. He was doing everything right, as best he knew: He got his refills each month and took the capsule every day, despite lack of improvement in his stomach symptoms. Maybe his doctor explained the reason for the new drug and George just didn't hear it. Or he forgot what the doctor had said. Or maybe the doctor said nothing and simply gave him the prescription. Regardless of what led to George's situation, it is something I see often and is repeated by millions of people every day. Without knowing the reason for the medication and how to measure if it is helping or not, George did not know when to follow up with his doctor about the new medicine or to question the benefit of continuing it for months on end. After meeting with me, George talked with his doctor, who stopped the omeprazole and evaluated other causes of his symptoms.

For George, the stomach medicine prescribed for him was not the solution to his problem. It was not effective, and he had to deal with the costs of that drug therapy. The costs included not only the price of the prescription each month, but also his time and effort to take the capsule each day, as well as the risk of possible side effects. Continuous use of omeprazole for months or years is associated with possible adverse effects such as bone fracture, low magnesium levels, and infection-related diarrhea.[1]

Too often, I see individuals who take their medicines for granted. Whether prescribed by their doctors or a product they take on their own, people assume the medication will be uniformly effective and without harm. Unfortunately, you probably do not have to look farther than a friend, relative, or the news to hear a story about an adverse drug event that led to a scary health encounter or even death. The drawbacks of improper use of medications are many, as will be discussed throughout this book. The ultimate challenge is for individuals who take medications to take only what is truly needed and effective for their situation, while avoiding drugs that are harmful and unnecessary. While not every adverse drug effect can be avoided, many of them can be prevented. The material in the following chapters opens the doors to understanding what improper use of medications looks like, how problems and errors arise, and steps that individuals can take to do something about the medication-use problem in America. While no age group is immune to this problem, the burden falls largely on the older adult population. To understand why this is so, it is important to take a moment to get a little background on the state of our aging nation.

THE AGING BOOM, MEDICATION USE, AND HEALTH-CARE COSTS

The US population is aging at an unprecedented rate. In medicine, the definition of "older adult" is anyone age sixty-five and older, and this age group is growing at a rate that far outpaces all others. Over the past ten years, the number of people younger than age sixty-five increased by 2 percent. This stands in contrast with a growth rate of 38 percent for individuals age sixty-five and older, and an even faster growth rate seen in-those age eighty-five and older. What about the number of persons a hundred years and older, you might ask? You guessed it; our centenarian population continues to climb each year, as well.[2] Another commonly cited statistic is that ten thousand Baby Boomers—individuals born between 1946 and 1964—are turning sixty-five every day through 2029.[3] All this growth translates to a swelling of the proportion of older adults in our population; it is expected to increase from 17 percent in 2022 to 22 percent in 2040.[4] These are a lot of data, and the numbers can be mind-numbing. But here is the key takeaway: we are in the midst of an unprecedented aging of our population. In turn, this tremendous growth has looming impact on the related concerns of medication use and health-care costs.

Aging goes hand-in-hand with medication use. From a pharmacy perspective, the projected growth in the number of older adults is alarming because they are most vulnerable to adverse drug events. Again, bear with me on some data: based on national health statistics, 89 percent of older adults take at least one prescription medication on a regular basis, while 42 percent take five or more.[5] The key takeaway here is that an increase in the sheer number of people who receive medications regularly lays the foundation for a potentially dangerous situation that cannot be ignored when it comes to medication safety.

Aging also is directly associated with higher health-care costs. These costs result from events such as more frequent doctor visits, use of home health care, emergency department visits, and hospitalizations.[6] Indeed, data show that overall costs for older adults are three times higher compared to those younger than sixty-five years.[7,8] As expected, the carve-out of medication costs parallels overall health-care dollars. Medication expenditures for older adults are significantly higher compared to younger age groups. According to David Lassman and colleagues, older adults spend more than twice as much on prescription drugs compared to adults who are younger than sixty-five: $1,900 vs. $850 per year.[9]

COSTS OF ADVERSE EFFECTS AND SUBOPTIMAL MEDICATION USE

Clearly, older adults are major consumers of medications, but they also are the most vulnerable to adverse effects. Based on national surveillance data of fifty-eight emergency departments (EDs) in the United States, a study published in the *Journal of the American Medical Association* looked at ED visits that resulted from an adverse drug event. Researchers found that 35 percent of these ED visits occurred in individuals who were age sixty-five and older.[10] Recall that this age group makes up a much smaller proportion of the population, just 17 percent. Researchers also found that older adults were three times more likely to take a trip to the ED because of a medication compared to persons younger than age sixty-five; and they were seven times more likely to be hospitalized because of the adverse drug event.[11] To state this another way, older adults are more likely to experience a drug-related event that is serious enough to require an ED visit and to be hospitalized from it. If you consider the huge growth of the aging population and how it uses more medications, the significance starts to become clear.

In 2019, the United States spent $3.8 trillion on health care. This included services like doctor visits and hospitalizations, as well as medications.[12] An important but overlooked contributor to this number is indirect costs that are related to suboptimal medication use, namely adverse outcomes that arise from the overuse, underuse, and misuse of drug therapy. When medications are prescribed or used improperly, they can cause adverse effects that lead to downstream health-care costs that far exceed the purchase price of the drug itself. These costs largely are *avoidable* and include added use of services like emergency department visits, hospitalizations, and admissions to long-term care facilities. Other costs stem from unplanned outpatient visits to physicians and additional medications that are prescribed to resolve problems caused by the initial drug.

Suboptimal use of drug therapy is preventable, with an estimated annual cost in the United States of $528.4 billion. It is associated with an estimated 275,689 deaths per year.[13] To put this in perspective, in 2020, there were 696,962 deaths from heart disease, 602,350 from cancer, and 200,955 from accidents.[14] Excluding 350,000 deaths from COVID-19 in 2020, that would put deaths due to suboptimal medication use as the third leading cause of death in the United States. In older adults specifically, indirect costs associated with using potentially inappropriate medications is estimated at $7.2 billion each year.[15] This might seem like a small fraction compared to the $129 billion that Medicare spends on prescription drugs,[16] but it represents billions of dollars that are needlessly spent and millions of lives that are negatively impacted by medications. When looking at spiraling health-care costs, it is no longer enough to conclude simply that medication prices are too high and we need to rein them in. We need to come to terms with the vast costs associated with *how* those medications are being used.

OLDER ADULTS AS A SPECIAL POPULATION

Healthcare for older patients is complex. It requires clinicians to integrate the physical aspects of aging with each patient's unique emotional, social, and financial characteristics. Each older adult patient is uniquely shaped by a lifetime accumulation of health behaviors, social support, and personal preferences, as well as a specific combination of illnesses. Treating an older patient means treating the *whole* patient, not just an isolated medical diagnosis. Treatment decisions need to be person-centered, involve the patient in decision-making, and address not only the person's physiology, but also psychological and social attributes. As a result, each patient's drug therapy plan and response to medications will be different.

Just as children are a special population in medicine (pediatrics), so are older adults (geriatrics). Medication use needs to be viewed with a trained eye that understands the nuances of an older patient. A baby cannot be given the same dosage of a medication as a thirty-year-old. In the same way, dosages and side effect warnings that are based on data collected in adults over the age of eighteen cannot be blindly extended to people age sixty-five years and older. Certain medicines no longer are appropriate choices in an older population. Drugs that have few safety concerns in younger adults can become a hazard to someone with multiple health conditions and age-related physiologic changes.

Unfortunately, geriatric training is the exception rather than the rule, and we currently lack sufficient numbers of geriatric-trained health-care professionals.[17,18] Fewer than 3 percent of physicians and about 1.5 percent of pharmacists are geriatric certified.[19,20] As a result, many healthcare providers who work with older patients may lack adequate knowledge to manage this population, especially with regard to the medications. Geriatric specialists offer a measure of assurance to patients and healthcare payers that they have the necessary skills and knowledge to optimize health outcomes and reduce unnecessary or inappropriate care of aging patients.

Gerontology and geriatrics are similar terms, but the distinction is important in medicine (see **Sidebar 1-1**).[21] People often confuse the terms or use them interchangeably. Gerontology is the broad study of the biological, psychological, and social aspects of the aging process. A gerontologist is an expert in aging but may not necessarily have medical training. In contrast, geriatrics is the medical specialty that focuses on health and disease as we age. All geriatricians are licensed medical doctors who have undergone additional specialty training.

SIDEBAR 1-1. GERONTOLOGY VS. GERIATRICS

Gerontology is the study of aging and the physical, mental, and social changes of people as they age. The field of gerontology brings together professionals from various disciplines, including social workers, psychologists, and health-care professionals. A gerontologist is a person who is trained in the biology, psychology, and sociology of aging to better understand the unique multifaceted aspects of aging.[22]

In contrast, geriatrics is a medical specialty area like cardiology or ophthalmology. A geriatrician is a medical doctor who has received specialized training in the treatment of the health-care needs of older adults. Geriatric medicine extends beyond mere physical concerns and typically uses a team-based approach to patient care.

Continued

Geriatricians are trained to focus on the following five key areas known as the Geriatric 5Ms that are important to all patients as they age:[23]

1. **Mind:** maintain mental activity; address issues of dementia, delirium, and depression
2. **Mobility:** maintain ability to walk and function independently; address balance and prevent falls
3. **Medications:** optimize prescribing based on the individual patient's needs; reduce use of multiple medications and risk of harmful effects
4. **Multi-complexity:** help older adults manage multiple medical conditions and complex psychosocial situations
5. **Matters most:** individualize care to meet the goals and preferences—what matters most—for each patient

IMPROVING MEDICATION USE

Why this book—a book about pharmacy and older patients—and why now? From my experience as a pharmacist talking with patients about their medications, I see patients who have questions and concerns, but do not know where to go for information or answers. Many of the problems caused by medications in older adults can be prevented if patients become more engaged to understand and ask key questions about the medications they take. Simply trusting that the drugs aren't causing problems is not enough. With guidance you will gain from this book, you can find your voice with the health-care professionals on your team. My goal is to empower you to become your own advocate or the advocate of a loved one.

The perfect storm is arriving: An aging population with multiple chronic conditions for whom medication use continues to increase;

health-care costs that are a concern for individuals and policymakers; and limited training in geriatric care that contributes to suboptimal medication use. As a nation, we will continue to see increased numbers of costly medication-related problems among older adults if we do not intervene. The good news is that this storm is leading to major paradigm shifts in health care that include a focus on person-centered care and the value of active patient involvement. The importance of patients participating in their health care decisions has been recognized as a way to improve quality of care and health outcomes.[24] Medical experts are joining efforts to raise awareness of risks associated with increased medication use among older adults and the need for greater patient engagement (see **Sidebar 1-2**).[25,26,27,28] Efforts are underway to evaluate interventions that can be implemented on a large scale across healthcare systems and to educate healthcare providers. The bad news is that these are seismic shifts that take time.

SIDEBAR 1-2. PARADIGM SHIFTS IN HEALTH CARE SUPPORTING PATIENT INVOLVEMENT

Choosing Wisely Campaign[29]

- This program was started in 2012 by the American Board of Internal Medicine Foundation to encourage conversations between patients and physicians in an effort to reduce unnecessary care. Today, there are dozens of medical specialty-specific lists that serve as resources for both clinicians and patients. These lists empower patients to ask their physician questions about procedures and treatments—even medications—that might be unnecessary or even harmful. New lists continue to be added.

Continued

Agency for Healthcare Research and Quality (AHRQ)[30]

- This federal agency published a White Paper in 2014 focused on providing high-quality primary care services. It lists several core components of an effective primary care practice, one of which is the patient–health-care team partnership. In addition, it mentions "informed, activated" patients as an important component of the healthcare team, leading to improved outcomes.

The Lown Institute[31,32]

- The Lown Institute is a nonpartisan think tank that published a landmark report in 2019 describing the widespread problem and serious consequences of "medication overload." In 2020, it published a national action plan to address this problem. Together, these two reports serve to elevate awareness about the extent of the problems associated with excess medication use and to create change. One of its core principles is to foster conversations between patients and clinicians about unnecessary and potentially harmful use of medications.

Rather than wait for these changes to occur, individuals can make a difference today to avoid unnecessary drug therapy and adverse drug reactions. It starts with becoming informed about the kinds of risks associated with drug therapy as we get older and how to reduce those risks. An example that illustrates the importance of this principle lies with Nick and his wife Nora.

When Nick called me with concerns about Nora, he was aware that medications could be causing changes to Nora's memory. She was seventy-six years old and a retired school librarian; she was active in book club, co-managing their finances, and enjoying her grandchildren. However, signs of memory loss over the past six months were noticeable to Nick.

I identified three drugs in Nora's regimen that could negatively impact memory: a drug to reduce spasms in her gut, an anti-anxiety drug, and an over-the-counter (OTC) product for sleep. After receiving my evaluation, Nora stopped the OTC sleep product and focused on non-drug ways to get to sleep. Then she and Nick engaged her physicians—two were involved in prescribing the medicines in question—to address their concerns about potential adverse drug effects.

The gastroenterologist agreed to stop the anti-spasm drug (which Nora had said wasn't effective), but her psychiatrist was resistant to making changes to the anti-anxiety medicine. Some medicines are more clearly of low value, questionable benefit, or potentially harmful, and thus easy to decide to stop. Others might require more patient-physician discussion about drug risks and benefits and what matters most to the patient (person-centered care). While Nora and her physician continued to talk about her concerns with the anti-anxiety medication, at least she had eliminated two potentially harmful drugs and noticed some improvement in her memory. I am grateful that this couple felt empowered enough to proactively question the medications and seek guidance. Ultimately, this book is based on the premise that educated consumers become wise patients, and wise patients are empowered to take their medications more safely and effectively and work with their health-care team to achieve better health outcomes.

I believe it is important to not simply tell people *what* to do, but to help them understand *why* to do it. Thus, this book contains two types of material. The first is information that addresses the *why*. It is designed to fill the knowledge gap of what we do not know about aging and medication use. Readers will learn why medications affect us differently as the body ages, what types of drugs are considered higher risk in older adults, important differences between OTC products and dietary supplements, and the key role of non-drug treatments. Terms like "polypharmacy" and "medication adherence" will be explained, clarifying how each contributes to medication-related problems.

The second type of material addresses the *what*. It contains the practical information that answers the question, "Now that I am aware of the risks, what can I do about it?" It is the consumer's guide on how to take and use medications in a more safe and effective manner to prevent medication-related problems. These chapters provide specific suggestions to help you better manage medications and refills, follow the medication instructions, and safely choose nonprescription products, for example. Most importantly, they contain lists of recommendations and questions to ask your physician or pharmacist to optimize medication use and catch potential problems or errors early.

While the material in this book focuses on older adults, it largely is applicable to a patient of any age. Anyone involved with helping adults age independently will learn something of value, even health professionals who need a refresher on geriatric pharmacy issues. This book is needed now because patients, caregivers, and health-care professionals must be knowledgeable about how to safely and properly use drug therapy in older adults. As individuals and stewards of our bodies, we need to understand how to use medications to maximize health and understand the serious nature of harms that can result when we misuse medications or take them carelessly. This book serves to foster awareness about the scope of medication-related problems and how to prevent them.

We must never take for granted the expectations placed on individuals to follow drug regimen instructions and modify behaviors that impact their health. Older adults who take multiple medications need to be followed and supported, but the risks of falling through the cracks in our health-care system pose a real threat. When these individuals carry the responsibility for managing multiple health problems and medications on their own, chances are high that something inadvertently will be neglected or overlooked. And when it is, the consequences can be great.

SUMMARY

Medication use is rampant and costly. Rather than simply taking medications because they are easily available and promise to fix our health woes, we need to be accountable for the medications we use. We do ourselves a disservice otherwise. As a society and individually, we must make a move to improve health outcomes. If we wait for the health-care system to fix the problems with how we use medications, we will remain at risk as consumers of drug therapy. However, if we learn how to work with our health-care team to be more mindful about medication use in older adults—in ourselves—and prevent medication-related problems, we can start correcting those problems today.

KEY POINTS

- Older adults are a growing segment of the US population; they have more chronic health conditions and rely more heavily on medications compared to younger patients.
- Older adults are at greater risk of experiencing medication-related problems, which contributes to increased health-care costs, suboptimal health outcomes, and reduced quality of life.
- Costs associated with suboptimal use of medications add a substantial burden to our health-care system and are avoidable.
- To reduce the risks of medication-related problems, we need to be more accountable about medication use in older adults at both a societal and individual level and seek more careful use of medications.

Chapter 2

Why Older Adults Are Vulnerable to Adverse Drug Events

Medication use carries more risk in older adults compared to younger individuals. While there is nothing magical about turning sixty-five years old, it is the minimum age that defines "older adult" and "geriatrics" in medicine. Thus, when talking about physiologic changes in the body and other health-related issues, pharmaceutical or medical, sixty-five signals the age at which, based on the chronologic clock, it is more common to see the onset of new health issues, changes in a person's susceptibility and response to illness, and of course, changes in how the body handles and responds to medications. This chapter begins to unpack the *Why* behind older adults being more vulnerable to adverse drug events. I boil it down to five characteristics common to older adults that collectively make this age group a high-risk population with regards to medication use (**Figure 2-1**).

By taking a moment to understand these factors that place older adults at greater risk of medication problems, you will be better able to take action to prevent problems in the longer-term. Knowledge is power. The majority of problems that older adults experience from their medications are preventable. This is key. But you first have to know what the causes are to know how to prevent them. Knowing the *Why* is the foundation for all that follows. It will be helpful in later chapters, for example when

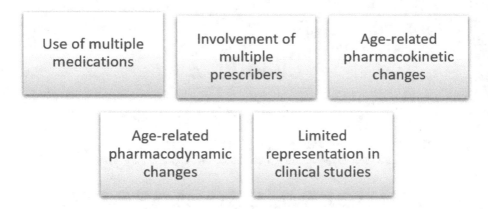

Figure 2-1. Five Characteristics that Increase the Risk of Adverse Drug Events in Older Adults

I talk about high-risk medications or the risk of serious consequences of drug interactions. As a result, you will better understand the rationale behind the guidance I have compiled, which will lead you to be more confident and comfortable to intervene with your health-care team and achieve safer, more appropriate medication use.

USE OF MULTIPLE MEDICATIONS

The older adult age group disproportionately consumes medications. While about 17 percent of the US population today is age sixty-five and older,[33] it accounts for an estimated 30 percent of drug expenditures.[34] This statistic directly reflects the greater presence of chronic health conditions in older individuals; more health conditions typically require more medications. The percentage of adults age sixty-five and older who take five or more prescription drugs continues to increase over time. It has tripled from 14 percent in 1988 to 42 percent in 2018.[35] Nearly 90 percent of older adults take at least one medication regularly.[36] The upward trend in medication use is alarming.

Taking multiple medications on a regular basis places older adults at an increased risk of experiencing a range of medication-related problems, such as drug interactions, adverse drug reactions (side effects), and the use of duplicated or unnecessary medications. Costs of taking multiple medications add up and can lead to more problems when affordability becomes an issue. Finally, as more medications are added to a person's list, the medication regimen can become complex. Older adults must remember to take each medication, take it correctly, and keep track of refills, for example. I frequently see patients who navigate not only taking medicines three or even four times a day, but they also have to remember to take certain ones before eating and others with food, plus master the proper technique for using inhalers, eye drops, and even an injectable medicine.

MULTIPLE PHYSICIANS PRESCRIBING

With age and additional health problems, it is common to have more than one doctor involved in one's care. I have heard many older adults joke about how their days are filled with doctor appointments. Indeed, more than half of older adults see two or more prescribers—physicians or other health-care professionals who prescribe medications for a person's care.[37] Individuals in this age group have an average of five chronic health conditions with three physicians prescribing medications for them,[38] and 10 percent have four or more prescribers involved in their care.[39] Fragmented care and involvement of multiple physicians are on the rise. Between 2000 and 2019, the proportion of Medicare beneficiaries who saw five or more specialist physicians increased from 17 to 30 percent.[40]

One of my clients had six physicians prescribing the medications in her regimen. Her husband was particularly eager to have my involvement because he knew the doctors were not in communication with each other. This client was feeling extremely tired throughout the day and had decreased memory that was of concern to her and her husband. Sure enough, I identified five medications that could cause sedation or drowsiness as well as negatively affect memory. I communicated this information to her physicians, drawing attention to the combination of medications that four different doctors were prescribing for her.

As this example illustrates, an increased number of physicians pre-scribing for an individual is associated with an increased risk of adverse drug events,[41] use of unnecessary medications,[42] and more difficulty in taking medications as instructed.[43,44] In fact, each additional prescriber increases the chance of having an adverse drug event by 29 percent.[45] Experts point to the lack of coordinated care between providers as the source of these problems, which is exactly what my client's husband had observed of his wife's care. In addition, lack of communication between physicians can lead to disjointed approaches to treating a medical condi-tion, with patients getting mixed messages and feeling overwhelmed.

I remember the first time a physician contacted me after reading my report, upset to learn that his patient was taking two medications that reduced acid production in the stomach. The patient was taking both omeprazole and lansoprazole—both proton pump inhibitors drugs, com-monly referred to by the abbreviation "PPI"—prescribed by both the pri-mary care doctor and a gastroenterologist (stomach specialist) and clearly an inappropriate duplication of therapy. The primary care physician on the phone insisted that I must be wrong. Once I explained that I had been in his patient's home, and the patient had shown me exactly what he was taking, the physician grew silent and changed his tone. The lack of care coordination between my client's prescribers was clear.

PHARMACOKINETIC CHANGES—CHANGES IN HOW THE BODY HANDLES MEDICATIONS

The word pharmacokinetics comes from the roots "pharmaco," meaning drugs, and "kinetics," meaning movement. Pharmacokinetics is the sci-ence of how drugs are handled by the body, or in other words, how drugs move through and are processed by the body. There are four components to the pharmacokinetic process, as depicted in **Figure 2-2**: absorption, distribution, metabolism, and elimination. These components, or stages, of pharmacokinetics describe the journey of a drug from when it is intro-duced into the body to when it is eventually eliminated from the body. Every drug has its own unique characteristics of what that journey looks

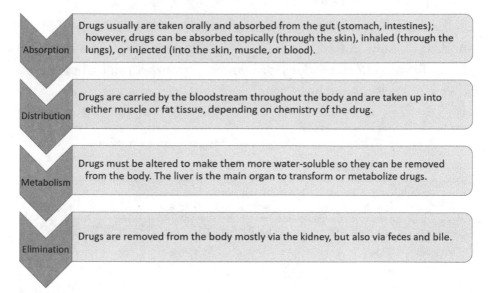

Figure 2-2. Four Components of Pharmacokinetics

like. In turn, these characteristics create a fairly predictable picture of the medication that enables clinicians to know how to safely use—or in some cases avoid—that medication for a particular patient. Pharmacokinetics forms the basis for understanding how to safely and properly dose and monitor medications, a central piece of pharmacists' expertise.

It is important to understand that with age, the body changes how it handles many medications. In other words, pharmacokinetics can be altered in older adults. Drug absorption, distribution, metabolism, and elimination can be impacted by the normal aging process. Key age-related changes are summarized in **Table 2-1**, along with common examples.[46,47] These changes predispose older adults to experiencing adverse drug events. Alterations to the components of metabolism and elimination generally pose greater risk than do changes that affect absorption and distribution of drugs. Reduced ability of the liver to transform or metabolize a medication can lead to a longer duration of action in the body. In turn, this increases the risk of side effects. Similarly, reduced kidney function causes slower elimination from the body of certain drugs and thus accumulation of those drugs and increased potential for side effects. To avoid either of these problems, prescribers can reduce medication doses or choose different drug therapy. Indeed, not reducing medication dosage with impaired kidney function in older adults is a common error that can lead to serious adverse drug events and hospitalization.[48,49]

Table 2-1. Age-Related Pharmacokinetic Changes Commonly Seen and Impact on Medication in Older Adults

Pharma-cokinetic component	Common changes with age	Impact on medications in older adults	Selected examples (not complete listing)
Absorption	Slowed gastric emptying Mild decrease in stomach acid production	Can lead to higher drug levels because of increased absorption. Some drugs might have reduced absorption because of reduced acid production, making them less effective.	Reduced absorption of vitamin B_{12}, iron, ketoconazole.
Distribu-tion	Decreased lean muscle mass Shift in body composition: increased body fat and decreased total water	Some medications have a greater than anticipated affect because of the shift in fat and water content. Others are eliminated more slowly from the body and have a prolonged effect.	Increased levels of digoxin, lithium, alcohol. Longer duration of activity and slower elimination of diazepam

Metabo-lism	Decreased size of and blood flow to liver Decreased ability to metabolize (transform) drugs	Can lead to higher or lower levels of medications, depending on the drug. More commonly, medications that rely on the liver to be metabolized are eliminated more slowly from the body and thus have higher risk of adverse effects.	Longer duration of activity of alprazolam, citalopram, diazepam, naproxen, sertraline, zolpidem Increased levels of diltiazem and verapamil
Elimina-tion	Decreased size of and blood flow to kidney Reduced ability to remove drugs from the body	Medications that rely on the kidneys to be removed from the body will have higher risk of adverse effects.	Slower elimination and longer time in the body of digoxin, famotidine, gabapentin, non-steroidal anti-inflammatory drugs (NSAIDs)

The good news is that adverse effects stemming from age-related changes in pharmacokinetics largely are preventable. When we have pharmacokinetic information for medications, combined with a patient's medical information, we can make adjustments to the medications to circumvent or avoid potential problems or, in some cases, simply monitor more carefully to reduce the risk of developing an adverse outcome.

PHARMACODYNAMIC CHANGES—CHANGES IN HOW MEDICATIONS AFFECT THE BODY

The word pharmacodynamics comes from the roots "pharmaco," meaning drugs, and "dynamics," meaning a pattern of activity. Pharmacodynamics is the science of the body's response to a drug or, in other words, how the drug affects the body. For example, blood pressure medications have certain actions (referred to as their "mechanisms of action") at specific targets in the body that lead to a decrease in blood pressure. Different drug classes have different targets. To use the example of two different classes of blood pressure medications, beta-blockers inhibit the activity of beta receptors that are located in blood vessels and the heart muscle, while the drug class of calcium-channel blockers works at a different target, namely, calcium channels.

There are multiple ways pharmacodynamics change with age. Various drug targets can become less sensitive, more sensitive, or reduced in number, for example. Another significant change is that drug molecules can more easily cross into the brain (that is, into the central nervous system). This means that with age, there is a much greater risk of adverse drug reactions like drowsiness, dizziness, decreased memory, and confusion that normally is not seen in younger persons.[50,51] The overall clinical impact is that individuals become more sensitive to the effects of medications with age, despite being exposed to "usual" or "normal" amounts of a drug. Pharmacodynamic changes are challenging to study and tend to be more variable from patient to patient. **Table 2-2** provides examples of common medications that are impacted by pharmacodynamic changes with increasing age. It is important to note that these medicines are still safe for older adults; they just might require more careful dosing and monitoring for effectiveness and side effects.

Table 2-2. Examples of Medications Impacted by Age-Related Pharmacodynamic Changes[52,53]

Example drug or drug class	Description of pharmacodynamic change common with aging
Warfarin:	Older adults are more sensitive to the effects of warfarin (a medication that reduces the ability of the blood to form blood clots), and starting doses for patients sixty-five years and older are one-half of those used in younger patients.

Sleep medicines and antidepressants:	Older adults are more sensitive to the sedating effects of sleep and depression medications; thus, lower starting doses are appropriate with gradual dose increases to give the body time to adjust and react to both the clinical (desired) and adverse effects of the medication.
Blood pressure medicines:	Older adults might be more sensitive to effects of blood pressure medicines and experience dizziness, especially when standing up quickly. This is because sensors in blood vessels react more slowly with age leading to a decrease in blood pressure; the blood vessels need more time to adjust and maintain blood pressure.

A common phrase in geriatric medicine is "start low, go slow." "Start low" refers to the need to begin with low doses of a medication to anticipate an increased sensitivity to both its clinical (desirable) and adverse effects. Older adults often respond to lower doses compared to doses that are prescribed for a general adult population. "Go slow" refers to the need to increase the dose gradually, giving the drug time to come to an equilibrium in the body and to allow for possible side effects to emerge. It is not uncommon for a reasonable starting dose in older adults to be 50 percent of the manufacturer's recommended starting dose.

Age-related pharmacodynamic changes are important because they can result in adverse drug reactions that are fairly subtle and may not be easily recognized as being caused by the medication. An older adult might experience a side effect or an exaggerated response to a medicine despite taking a "usual" dose because of greater sensitivity in the body. Clinicians who are not alert to the potential for an exaggerated response may start older patients at doses that would be appropriate for the general adult population, but that are too high for older individuals. Similarly, the dose might be increased too quickly and lead to adverse effects.

There are several important examples of increased sensitivity to a drug's effects. Use of the blood thinner warfarin (Coumadin®) can lead to serious bleeding events if given to older adults at the "usual" recommended dosage. Blood pressure medicines like metoprolol or lisinopril often are started at very low doses to reduce the potential for side effects. Similarly, many drugs that act within the brain are effective at low initial doses for older individuals. They can be increased slowly, if needed, as long as the patient is not having side effects. The mantra "start low, go slow" accounts for pharmacodynamic changes and helps maximize the benefit of a medication while avoiding unwanted effects.

LIMITED REPRESENTATION IN CLINICAL STUDIES

To learn about the effects of a drug in a special population like geriatrics, the drug must be studied in that population. Physiologic changes (such as the pharmacokinetic and pharmacodynamic effects discussed previously) that occur with aging mean that we cannot assume a medication will behave the same way in older patients as it does in younger adults. Unfortunately, older adults frequently are excluded from clinical trials or not represented in large enough numbers. Inclusion of older adults is important during the clinical research phase of a drug's life cycle because it helps to detect adverse events, as described in **Sidebar 2-1**.

SIDEBAR 2-1. DETECTING ADVERSE EVENTS IN CLINICAL STUDIES

The FDA regulates all drugs in the United States and mandates rigorous clinical studies to document safety and effectiveness of each medication prior to federal approval. This is done through premarketing studies, which occur in three phases. Phase 1 studies enroll twenty to a hundred healthy volunteers to study the safety of a drug in humans.

Phase 2 studies typically enroll forty to 300 patients with a focus on the drug's effectiveness, along with continued safety evaluation. Finally, Phase 3 studies enroll anywhere from dozens to a few thousand patients. By the time an investigational drug is submitted to the FDA for approval, it has been tested in maybe 3000 to 4000 patients. This is a tiny number of people compared to the millions who will be exposed to the medication after it is approved. The small number of exposures allows for detection only of fairly common adverse events; namely, events that occur in from one to five out of a hundred persons. There is an 80 percent to 99 percent chance that common adverse events will be detected before a drug is approved. More rare events that occur in only one out of 1000 people or less frequently, however, have less than a 7 percent chance of being detected in a sample of 3000 or 4000 patients.[54,55]

Typically, clinical trials include from only a few dozen to a few hundred older adults. Enrollment of participants who are age seventy-five and above is even smaller. For example, the diabetes drug sitagliptin (Januvia®) was studied in 725 individuals age sixty-five and older and only sixty-one persons age seventy-five and above. Prucalopride (Motegrity®) was approved in 2018 for treating constipation. It was studied in 372 persons sixty-five and older and in 124 persons seventy-five and older.[56,57]

For most newly approved medications, issues of concern specific to older adults cannot be known until once the drug is approved and widely prescribed. It is estimated that it can take five to ten years to identify significant adverse effects. Therefore, it is reasonable to wait until a medication has been on the market for at least a few years to allow time to uncover more information about the safety of a medication before prescribing it in older adults.[58,59]

Many older adults are medically complex—they have multiple health conditions and take multiple medications. Including these more complex patients in clinical research is challenging because it makes it harder for researchers to isolate the effect of the new investigational drug when other health conditions or medications also are present. In addition, there are perceived safety issues when testing a new drug in older participants who might be in poorer health. However, without studying a drug in "real-world" individuals who have other health conditions and take other medications at the same time, we lack data on safety and effectiveness once the drug gets approved.[60] National initiatives have encouraged enrollment of older adults in clinical trials to address the lack of representation in studies. In 1993, the Food and Drug Administration (FDA) issued a guideline for pharmaceutical manufacturers recommending that older adults be included in the studies of drugs anticipated to have significant use in older adults.[61] In 2019, the National Institutes of Health (NIH) initiated "Inclusion Across the Lifespan," a policy to encourage inclusion of pediatric and geriatric patients in NIH-sponsored trials as appropriate. The program focuses on the need to include patients in clinical trials who ultimately will take and benefit from the treatment being studied.[62]

Despite these efforts, many older adults remain unable to enroll in clinical trials. One report found that 28 percent of research trials excluded older adults.[63] The downstream impact of having limited representation in clinical research is that there is insufficient information to guide healthcare providers on how to safely use a medication in that population. Information from clinical trials eventually is summarized by the pharmaceutical manufacturer and included in what is referred to as a drug's Product Information, or labeling information, which becomes a key resource for clinicians.

The Product Information is a standardized document required by the FDA for every approved drug. However, studies evaluating the content of this information have found that data regarding use in geriatric patients frequently are lacking. One study found that only 33 percent of 214 newly approved medications had sufficient information to guide geriatric use.[64] Another study reviewed forty-two newly approved drugs and found that

57 percent of the Product Information material addressed dosing and/or safety in older adults.[65] In other words, based on these studies, roughly half (43 percent to 67 percent) of drugs approved by the FDA lack sufficient information to guide prescribing in geriatric patients.

PROTECTING AGAINST THESE RISKS

The five factors discussed in this chapter taken together are unique to older adults and create an environment that makes this age group more vulnerable to adverse drug events. At first glance, it might appear that these factors are largely beyond our control. However, knowledge is power. Knowledge of these factors—understanding the *Why*—empowers older adults to be proactive with their healthcare team and take steps to reduce the chance that medications will cause a serious problem. What can individuals do—what can *you* do—to protect against these factors?

1. Recognize that you are a member of your healthcare team. You have an active voice to discuss and ask questions about choices regarding how to manage your health, including medications. The concept of a healthcare team is described in more detail in **Sidebar 2-2**.

2. Focus on ways to reduce the number of medications you take. This might involve asking about non-drug ways to manage your health conditions, asking for a comprehensive medication review to identify duplicated or potentially unnecessary medications, and adopting healthy lifestyle habits to prevent new or worsened health conditions. These topics are discussed in more detail in other chapters.

3. If you see more than one physician, make sure they are in communication with each other, especially regarding your medication list. Have your primary care physician—or one of your physicians— oversee all of your care and help you resolve any contradictory health advice or complex instructions. If necessary, get a geriatric specialist involved.

4. To address concerns that can stem from pharmacokinetic changes with age, make sure you know about any changes in the health of your kidneys or liver. If you have kidney or liver impairment, you should be aware that it can impact drug dosages or choice of drug. Thus, if it applies to you, before starting a new medication, ask your physician or pharmacist if the drug is affected by changes in kidney or liver function. Ask your pharmacist if any of your medications need to have lower doses because of age-related changes in kidney function.

5. When a new medication is added, be alert to possible side effects. Ask your doctor if starting with a low dose might be warranted for you because of your age, kidney function, or other health conditions. Talk with your doctor about increasing doses slowly when needed, to give your body time to adjust and detect side effects.

6. Unless it is considered absolutely essential, avoid taking a newly approved medication until it has been on the market for a few years. Some experts recommend waiting at least five years to allow for rare adverse effects to be detected.[66]

SIDEBAR 2-2. THE HEALTH-CARE TEAM

Yes, you have a health-care team. It exists whenever you are a patient and receive care from a health-care professional. Who makes up your team? Think of everyone involved in the health care you receive:

- physician
- nurse
- pharmacist
- physical therapist
- occupational therapist
- dentist
- dietitian
- psychologist
- social worker
- patient

And there are still others you might include on your list. However, the most important member on any healthcare team is the last one listed: you, the patient. While you may not be aware of it, you are part of the decision-making process, and your preferences and observations matter. As such, you have the right to be part of the plans and decisions surrounding your care. The shift toward person-centered care has heightened this awareness.

While clinicians on your team are experts in the science, education, and evidence of safe and effective treatment options, you are the expert in what matters most to you, what you prioritize in life, and what makes you an individual. To successfully counter the factors that make older adults more vulnerable to adverse drug events means that you need to speak up on your healthcare team and raise questions to ensure that you take only the most appropriate drug therapy that benefits your health and priorities. We cannot move toward safer, more careful use of medications, without your voice as a member of your health-care team.

SUMMARY

There are five key factors that collectively shed light on why older adults are more vulnerable to experiencing adverse drug events compared to a younger adult population. As a result, we need to look at medication use a little differently in this population and be aware of the potential for various risks. Awareness of these factors allows individuals to make wiser choices with their healthcare team to optimize the benefits that medications offer while minimizing potential harm.

KEY POINTS

- Older adults are more susceptible to medication-related problems compared to the younger adult population because they take multiple medications, they often have more than one prescriber involved in their care, they experience age-related physiologic changes (pharmacokinetic and pharmacodynamic changes), and they are often under-represented in clinical research trials.
- Older adults need to be viewed as a unique population with regard to medication use because they are more vulnerable to experiencing an adverse drug event.
- Individuals can use this information to be more engaged as part of their health-care team to optimize the benefits that medications offer while minimizing potential harm.

Chapter 3

Understanding Medication-Related Problems and Medication Reviews

If I had a dime for every time I heard someone tell me, "I don't need a medication review; I only take what my doctor tells me to take," I would be a rich woman, as the saying goes. Many people tend to take their medications for granted and assume nothing can go wrong. Indeed, there is a wide margin of safety for most of the prescription drugs marketed today. However, when used in a "real world" setting, beyond the environment of a clinical trial, medications that pose minimal risk in younger and fairly healthy individuals might have a greater risk of harm in older adults. As described in the previous chapter, individuals age sixty-five and older are at increased risk of experiencing adverse drug effects. Moreover, interactions with other drugs and health conditions, as described in later chapters, further complicate the picture of drug safety and appropriateness. Just because an individual "takes only what the doctor prescribes," it does not guarantee protection against adverse effects. If it were that simple, we would not see emergency department visits and hospitalizations resulting from medication use. And while a physician might have a list of each patient's prescribed medications, this, too, cannot guarantee the absence of problems. A medication list is like the hood of a car. The car might look good on the surface, but you need to check under the hood to really know if the car is in good working condition. The difficult truth is that problems can and do arise, despite the best efforts to prescribe drugs that will be safe and effective.

I once had a phone conversation with the niece and guardian of a seventy-eight-year-old woman who was prescribed fifteen medications. The aunt was referred to me by a social worker for a medication review. The niece expressed to the social worker various concerns about her aunt's health and other stressors she had as a caregiver. Notably, her aunt had become very unsteady and lethargic and was not consistently taking her medicines. She was at high risk for a fall. The social worker recognized the potential for medication side effects and knew that I could also help the niece understand more about the medicines her aunt was taking, help her to more easily manage her aunt's medications day-to-day, and assist her in communicating about medication concerns and side effects to the doctors. Based on the criteria for a citywide program at the time, the aunt was eligible for a medication review at no charge. Yet the niece had no interest. She readily justified to me why her aunt was not at risk of having a medication-related problem and did not need the review: "She only takes what the doctor prescribes; plus, she sees three different doctors regularly, and they all look at her medications." She spoke with assurance, her tone questioning the value of a medication review. She was certain that because the physicians were aware of her aunt's medication list, her aunt must be sufficiently protected. The niece did not recognize how her aunt's medications indeed could be contributing not only to her aunt's symptoms and fall risk, but also to her own stress as she tried to manage a complex and unfamiliar medicine list.

The niece, along with many people, are hesitant to recognize that medications can lead to unanticipated problems, but why is this? Part of the reason consumers might be over-confident in the safety of their medications stems from misconceptions about the role of the FDA in regulating drugs. A survey published online in 2019 in the journal *Pharmacoepidemiology and Drug Safety* found that a slight majority (57 percent) of respondents correctly knew that the FDA approves drugs when the benefits are greater than its risks.[67] However, 23 percent of respondents falsely believed that drugs approved by the FDA will not cause harm. Yes, there is a level of safety for FDA-approved medications; but all drugs carry the potential for adverse events. Very few medications, if any, are totally risk free. Using a medication involves weighing the potential for good against the potential negative effects or harms. In most cases, the good outweighs the bad. But this is not always the case, which is why extra care sometimes is needed.

There are many facets that make up the big picture of appropriate medication use. Taking only what your doctor prescribes is one facet. However, it misses other critical and sometimes less obvious problems that can undermine the safety and effectiveness of medications. A medication list might seem appropriate when a clinician first glances at it, but looking more closely—checking under the hood for the types of medication-related problems that are described in this chapter—provides a more complete picture of potential pitfalls in a drug regimen and helps to prevent problems from occurring.

This chapter digs a little deeper into the nature of adverse drug events. It introduces the concept of medication-related problems (MRPs), which is the starting place from where we can improve the safety and effectiveness of medication use. While not all MRPs are obvious to the consumer, most are preventable. Identifying MRPs is key to reducing undesirable downstream effects. With a solid understanding of the broad scope and nature of these problems, you can better appreciate the value of a medication review and how it helps you, your physician, and your pharmacist identify and avoid many MRPs.

EIGHT CATEGORIES OF MEDICATION-RELATED PROBLEMS

A MRP is defined as an event involving medication therapy that actually or potentially gets in the way of a desired health outcome. An important part of this definition is that the problem can be a potential concern—it has not yet occurred—or it can be a problem that already is present. It is worth noting that even an actual MRP may not always lead to a noticeable issue for a patient; however, many can and do cause adverse events. Ideally, MRPs can be identified when they still are potential issues and can thus be corrected before leading to a negative health outcome. MRPs commonly are grouped into eight categories as described in **Table 3-1**.[68]

Table 3-1. Eight Categories of Medication-Related Problems[69]

Category	Description	Example
1. Adverse drug reactions	The patient experiences a side effect or other unwanted or unexpected response to a medication.	A patient experiences nausea and vomiting caused by metformin (Glucophage®).
2. Drug interactions	The patient is taking a medication that inter-acts with another drug, medical condition, food, or alcohol.	A patient is taking the blood thinner apixaban (Eliquis®) and self-medicates with over-the-counter ibuprofen for arthritis pain. The interaction between the blood thinner and ibuprofen can lead to a serious bleeding event.
3. Dose that is too low	The patient is taking a dose that is too low and is not clinically effective.	A patient who is taking lisino-pril (Zestril®) 5 mg daily to treat hypertension, but blood pressure still is too high.
4. Dose that is too high	The patient is taking a dose that is too high based on recommended dosing guidelines or indi-vidual characteristics like age, other medications, or health conditions.	A patient has impaired kidney function and is taking a medica-tion that relies on the kidney for elimination at full (usual) dose; the dose needs to be reduced to avoid side effects.

5. Selection of improper drug	The patient is taking a medication that is either not effective for the condition or is not appropriate for the patient based on age, interactions, or adverse effect potential (risks are greater than benefit).	An older adult is taking diazepam (Valium®) at bedtime every night for sleep, thus increasing the risk of a fall and hip fracture, decreased memory, and confusion. Other treatment options would be safer.
6. Untreated or under-treated condition	The patient has a medical condition but is not being treated for it or it is only partially treated (undertreatment).	A patient had low levels of vitamin D and is told to buy a vitamin D supplement but never does.
7. Not receiving a medication	The patient is not taking a medication that he should be taking (drug therapy has been prescribed).	A patient never gets a new medication filled. A patient does not know how to correctly use his inhaler to treat his breathing condition; he has shortness of breath because the medication is not getting into his lungs.
8. Unnecessary medications	The patient is taking a medication that has no medical reason (indication), is no longer effective, or is a duplication of therapy.	A patient was started on omeprazole during a hospital stay, but it was mistakenly continued once the patient was discharged to home and there is no longer a clinical reason for it.

To illustrate each category, let me borrow a medication list from my client Francis that reflects the regimens of many of my clients.

- Amlodipine (Norvasc®) 15 mg once daily to treat high blood pressure (hypertension)
- Furosemide (Lasix®) 20 mg once daily to treat fluid retention (ankle swelling)
- Gabapentin (Neurontin®) 300 mg once daily in the evening for nerve pain in the feet
- Latanoprost (Xalatan®) eye drops, one drop in each eye daily at bedtime to treat glaucoma
- Simvastatin (Zocor®) 40 mg once daily in the evening to lower cholesterol
- Tolterodine LA (Detrol LA®) 4 mg, once daily to treat overactive bladder
- Trazodone (Desyrel®) 50 mg once daily at bedtime (this is an antidepressant at higher doses, but it is prescribed at low doses for sleep because it causes drowsiness)
- Zolpidem (Ambien®) 5 mg once daily at bedtime for sleep

Adverse Drug Reactions. The first type of MRP is adverse drug reactions. After reviewing Francis's medications and speaking with her about her health conditions, symptoms, and when her different medications were started, it was uncovered that amlodipine was causing fluid retention in her ankles. This led to her doctor adding a diuretic (water pill) furosemide about two months after the dose of amlodipine was increased. I noticed another adverse drug reaction that was a side effect of tolterodine: in listening to Francis speak, it was clear she had dry mouth. When I asked her about it, she recalled that it started around the time she began taking tolterodine to treat her incontinence episodes. Bingo; common side effects of tolterodine and related medicines for treating overactive bladder are dry mouth and dry eyes. She said she had never thought about mentioning it to her doctor, and her doctor never asked. Francis never put two and two together and may never have known that her dry mouth was a drug side effect.

Drug Interactions. The second category, drug interactions, is illustrated in a few different ways. First, amlodipine and simvastatin interact. Combining these two medicines can lead to increased blood levels of simvastatin and a higher chance of side effects from it. As a result, when these drugs are used together, the simvastatin dose should be reduced to manage the interaction and limit the risk of an adverse drug reaction. Zolpidem, gabapentin, and trazodone provide another example of drugs that interact. In this case, all three medicines have a central "mechanism of action" (that is, they work in the brain). When taken in combination, there is the increased chance of experiencing side effects such as sedation, dizziness, and fall risk. The interaction can be clinically important and needs to be watched for carefully. Similarly, the combination of tolterodine and trazodone can increase the chance of side effects like dry mouth that Francis had, dry eyes, blurred vision, and constipation. The combination can also increase the potential for impaired memory and confusion, which is of particular concern in older adults. Drug interactions are discussed in more detail in Chapter 9.

Dose That Is Too Low. Gabapentin illustrates the third type of problem, a dose that is too low. Francis's doctor prescribed this medication six months earlier after discussing a new symptom of tingling in her feet. She has not noticed any change in her symptoms but her dose may be too low to be effective. A starting dose of gabapentin 300 mg at bedtime is commonly prescribed to minimize the risk of side effects; however, the effective dose of gabapentin for treating nerve pain is 1800 to 3600 mg per day. Thus, it is quite likely that Francis's dose of gabapentin needs to be increased gradually to a therapeutic dose of at least 600 mg three times a day, as long as she does not have side effects.

Dose That Is Too High. Francis's dose of amlodipine illustrates the fourth type of MRP, which is the problem of having a dose that is too high. The maximum recommended dose of amlodipine is 10 mg per day. Thus, taking a dose of 15 mg increases her risk of side effects, such as fluid retention in the ankles. Lowering the dose of amlodipine likely will reduce or reverse this side effect; possibly amlodipine might need to be switched to a different blood pressure medicine, as well.

Improper Drug Selection. The fifth category of MRPs is selection of an improper drug. In Francis's regimen, zolpidem illustrates this type of problem. Zolpidem is one of a number of medications that are considered to be potentially inappropriate in older adults, as will be discussed in Chapter 10. Zolpidem and other sedative-hypnotic drugs are not good choices because the risks are felt to outweigh benefits in older individuals. Specifically, zolpidem places Francis at increased risk of experiencing a fall and related fracture; it can affect her balance and contribute to next-day drowsiness. These risks are compounded by interactions with gabapentin and trazodone mentioned previously.

Untreated Condition. The sixth type of MRP is an untreated condition. Untreated conditions typically cannot be detected simply by looking over the list of medications a person takes. Generally, the pharmacist or other clinician who is reviewing a person's medications would need to get more information from the patient and review the person's medical record. In Francis's case, after speaking with her about her sleep pattern, I learned that she had been struggling with a very painful neck and shoulders that she attributed to arthritis and getting older. This pain interfered with her sleep, and for the past few months she had been trying over-the-counter products. She finally asked her doctor if there was a prescription drug that could help. This is when her doctor added zolpidem. Thus, her pain at night in particular was an important untreated condition. It even led to her being prescribed an additional medication, zolpidem. I recommended that Francis consider using oral acetaminophen or topical diclofenac gel to help with the pain. Her doctor spoke with her about seeing a physical therapist and also using cold and heat packs to provide additional relief. Once her pain control was improved, Francis was able to sleep better and no longer needed the zolpidem, but more on that soon.

Not Receiving a Medication. The seventh category of MRP, not receiving a medication, is pretty much impossible to detect by looking only at a medication list. Just because a medicine is prescribed for an individual does not mean that the medicine is being taken or taken correctly. This type of MRP can lead to medical problems that are untreated or undertreated, which in turn can cause worsened health outcomes. Once a medication is prescribed, it has to get into the body so it can have its intended clinical effect. Not receiving a medication can include anything from someone not taking a medicine because it is too expensive to a person inserting a suppository with the wrapper still on it that prevents it from being absorbed (this is a true story we were taught in pharmacy school!). Francis, I learned, was administering her glaucoma eye drop latanoprost incorrectly by placing the drop in her eye and then blinking so it ran down her cheek. She was not aware that this simply wasted the eye drop and made it useless for treating glaucoma. To be effective, there are a series of steps to properly place the drop in the eye and keep it there so it can be absorbed. I educated Francis about correct eye drop technique. In addition, her ophthalmologist needed to be informed of this unexpected delay in starting her glaucoma treatment, in case it could impact the doctor's follow-up assessment of the new drug's effectiveness. Not receiving a medication falls under the topic of medication adherence, discussed in Chapter 8.

Unnecessary Medication Use. The eighth category of MRPs is unnecessary medication use. This is perhaps one of the more important categories, in light of the overmedication problem we face in the United States. To me, identifying even one medication that an individual no longer needs and that can be stopped or reduced is a huge success. Once I dug deeper into Francis's medication regimen—looking under the hood, if you will—I uncovered several issues with her current medications that identified them as possibly unnecessary. Once her pain was better managed, both zolpidem and trazodone for sleep became unnecessary. She had been taking trazodone for years, but it had been of no benefit for quite a while and should have been stopped earlier. Once amlodipine was identified as the cause of ankle swelling, her physician lowered the dose, the ankle swelling improved, and furosemide was no longer needed, as well.

PREVENTION OF MEDICATION-RELATED PROBLEMS

MRPs matter because they are pervasive in our health-care system. They are estimated to cost $528.4 billion annually in the United States.[70] Compared to patients younger than age sixty-five, older adults are at least two times more likely to end up with an emergency department visit or a hospitalization caused by an adverse drug event.[71,72] In addition, 28 percent to 72 percent of medication-related hospital admissions are deemed to have been preventable.[73,74,75,76] Even if we conservatively estimate that more than one-quarter and likely somewhere around one-half of hospitalizations caused by an adverse drug event could have been prevented, that is a humbling statistic. These data reinforce the need to be proactive in identifying and addressing MRPs.

Knowing that MRPs are preventable, what can we do as consumers or as healthcare professionals to make a dent in the situation? Where and how can we intervene to prevent a MRP from developing? The following three areas are the most commonly identified as contributing to problems: prescribing issues and drug selection, drug therapy monitoring, and patient education.[77,78,79,80] You might already be thinking, "Okay, I see where I can get involved and learn more about my medications; but what can I do about prescribing issues or drug monitoring?" I agree—these two areas largely are the responsibility of your health-care providers. But recall, too, that identifying and preventing medication-related problems ideally is a team effort, and you are a key player on that team. Upcoming chapters in this book provide information, strategies, and questions you can ask that enable you to be more engaged even with prescribing issues and monitoring of your drug therapy.

Prescribing and drug selection involves choosing the right drug and the right dose for an older adult patient. It needs to factor in not only a person's age, but also changes in kidney and liver function that were discussed in the previous chapter, as well as the presence of interacting drugs and medical conditions. As a result of pharmacokinetic and pharmacodynamic changes with age, there are a number of medications that have been identified as potentially inappropriate and high-risk that need to be used more carefully. These drugs are discussed in Chapters 10 and 11.

Careful monitoring of drug therapy is essential. Monitoring means to observe or keep track of signs and symptoms over time. Medicines need to be regularly assessed for both desired and unwanted effects. Monitoring can involve blood tests that measure drug concentrations to ensure medicine dosages are safe and in the effective range. Or it can involve blood tests that track kidney and liver function to detect changes that could be caused by medications. Other ways to monitor drug therapy is to look for signs of effectiveness, such as by checking blood pressure, blood sugar level, or daily weight. Importantly, patients and their health-care providers need to be alert to new symptoms that could be drug side effects, such as a rash, nausea, dizziness, or more serious symptoms like shortness of breath or bleeding. Routine monitoring of drug therapy allows for problems to be detected—and hopefully detected early—so that changes can be made to avert a serious negative outcome.

Finally, patients need to have sufficient knowledge about their medications to take them properly and safely at home. Health-care professionals have a responsibility to educate patients about their health conditions, treatment options, and the medications prescribed. Pharmacists especially are trained to communicate with patients about drug therapy. Unfortunately, in our hurried and fragmented health-care system, these educational opportunities can be glossed over, rushed, or simply missed. As a result, individuals may not always get the information they need, which can increase the risk of MRPs.

PATIENT ROLE IN PREVENTING MEDICATION-RELATED PROBLEMS

While much of the responsibility for preventing MRPs justifiably lies with health-care professionals—to carefully select drug therapy, appropriately monitor it, and educate patients so drug therapy is taken properly at home—prevention of MRPs is a team sport and very much a two-way street. The material throughout this book helps to empower you to be pro-active as a patient and consumer. As described in Chapter 14, you should know basic information about each of your medications. If this informa-tion is not offered at the doctor's office or pharmacy, then be the squeaky wheel and ask. At minimum, know the reason for each drug and how to take it properly—whether this is knowing how many times a day to take it or knowing how to correctly use eye drops or an inhaler.

Follow the instructions for when and how to take your medications. Know what side effects to watch for and what to do if there is a problem. It also is important to know what to monitor and to follow through with these instructions. This might involve a trip to the lab for a blood test, keeping a daily diary at home, or being alert to side effects or a change in symptoms. Finally, the patient-pharmacist partnership can be invaluable to ensure you are well-informed about your drug therapy. Take advantage of the wealth of knowledge pharmacists have, and make the time to ask your pharmacist about each medication.

An important step you can take to defend against MRPs is to get a thorough review once a year. This is different than having someone "look over" your medications. A study published in 2018 in the *British Journal of Pharmacology* found that only 6 percent of MRPs could be identified by looking at the medication list without interviewing the patient as well.[81] Interviewing patients as part of a medication review was necessary to iden-tify the majority (84 percent) of problems. Thus, in the span of a brief office visit, it is unlikely that a clinician will uncover more than a few, if any, problems. A thorough review allows for a more critical and objective look to assess if medications are effective, causing a possible side effect, or are no longer needed, for example.

Too often I hear from clients, "My doctor knows all my medicines, so everything is fine," or "I asked my doctor to review my medication list, and he said everything is working fine; there's no need to change anything." MRPs frequently go unnoticed. My concern is that busy phy-sicians may not have the time to critically and objectively assess a patient's medications. I admit that I am biased because I know the value of a phar-macist's training. But I also have seen myriad problems that go undetected among older adults who live in the community and are doing their best to manage multiple medications on their own. Thus, consider the value of having a medication expert—ideally a pharmacist with geriatric expertise—objectively review your medications and look under the hood to identify actual or potential problems. **Sidebar 3-1** provides guidance to help determine who will most benefit from a medication review and how to find a pharmacist to provide one.

SIDEBAR 3-1. WHO CAN BENEFIT FROM A MEDICATION REVIEW?

Who is at greatest risk of experiencing a medication-related problem? Should every older adult have their medications reviewed by a geriatric pharmacist expert—also known as a senior care pharmacist? Ideally, it would be a wonderful safeguard for all older adults to have a review, but this is neither feasible nor practical. The next best option is to identify people who are at higher risk of experiencing an adverse drug event. Several characteristics have been identified that can contribute to a higher risk of an older adult experiencing a medication-related problem:[82,83]

- Taking five or more medications on a regular basis
- Having more than one physician prescribing medications on a regular basis
- Being treated for three or more medical problems
- Use of more than one pharmacy to obtain prescription medications
- Difficulty remembering to take medications
- Having a complex drug regimen, often defined as taking twelve or more doses per day (for example, taking a

Continued

medicine twice a day is two doses; taking a medicine three times a day is three doses, etc.)

- Taking medications that require different administration techniques (such as inhalers, eye drops, injectable drugs)
- Having frequent changes to the medication regimen or recent hospitalization
- Taking certain types of medications:
  - Drugs that need blood-level monitoring (these include carbamazepine, digoxin, lithium, phenytoin, and warfarin, among others)
  - Drugs that increase fall risk (these generally include antidepressants, benzodiazepines, antiepileptic medications, and opioid pain medicines)
  - Drugs that can cause low blood-sugar levels (these include insulin, glimepiride, glipizide, and glyburide, among others)

The more of these characteristics that someone has, the greater the chance is that the person might experience a medication-related problem. These individuals likely will benefit from a thorough medication review to identify and correct actual or potential problems. In addition, I encourage anyone who has questions about being overmedicated or side effects to seek a medication review.

Unfortunately, in our current health-care system, medication reviews are not universally available largely because of the lack of a consistent payment mechanism. Pharmacists may not always be available to provide this service, but I am optimistic this will change in the near future, as there is a growing recognition of the value of pharmacist involvement as part of a team-based approach to improve health outcomes. While I am biased toward the expertise that a pharmacist brings to the table, other health-care professionals who have expertise in geriatric drug therapy are a good resource for providing a medication review. Here are a few recommendations to guide you in finding a qualified pharmacist for a medication review.

Search for an independent consultant pharmacist (also called a senior care pharmacist) in your area. Senior care pharmacists are experts in geriatric drug therapy. While many provide clinical pharmacy services to nursing home residents, some have community-based practices where they offer medication reviews and other medication-management services. Check with trusted referral sources in your community, such as a local senior center, the Area Agency on Aging, or your physicians. They should be able to steer you in the right direction. Also, the American Society of Consultant Pharmacists has an online national Senior Care Pharmacist Directory to help find a senior care pharmacist in your state at the website HelpWithMyMeds. org (https://www.ascp.com/mpage/Care_Pharmacist).

Some of the larger medical clinics have part or full-time pharmacists on the medical team. Thus, ask if your physician's office has a pharmacist on staff. Also, ask at your community (retail) pharmacy. Your pharmacist there might provide medication reviews by appointment. If your current pharmacy does not have this service, ask around to see if another one does. Independent pharmacies might offer more personalized services that are not available at larger chains. And of course, contact your Medicare Part D plan to find out if you are eligible for an annual comprehensive medication review as described in Sidebar 3-2. These reviews are free of charge, but they are not always conducted in-person and might not be provided by a pharmacist.

WHAT TO EXPECT IN A MEDICATION REVIEW

What does a typical medication review look like, and what can you expect during the process? While there will be variations, certain components should be common to a medication review, which centers on the patient interview. You can expect the pharmacist to gather all of your medications and create a complete and accurate medication list. This will include prescription and nonprescription medications and those you take just occasionally or "as needed." You likely will be asked a series of questions that helps the pharmacist understand what you already know about your medications, if you feel they are helping you, and whether you are aware of any side effects. The pharmacist will want to know how you take each of your medications every day, if you use a pill organizer or another system to organize your medicines, how you typically remember when and how to take your medicines, and if you sometimes miss or forget doses. The pharmacist also might ask about how you get your refills each month.

Other questions might explore lifestyle topics like sleep or meal patterns and how much exercise or physical activity you get on a daily basis. Questions about use of tobacco, alcohol, and recreational drugs will be part of the review, too. In addition, pharmacists will assess for various potential or actual MRPs, identify goals of drug therapy, and evaluate appropriate choice of medications (drug selection) based on your age and specific health conditions.

Following the medication interview, the pharmacist will provide a written report that includes your medication list and the pharmacist's recommendations. The pharmacist also can help you simplify your medication schedule, if needed, so that your schedule is more manageable.

Be prepared that there might be a cost for a medication review. It is a common misunderstanding that pharmacists routinely can bill insurance companies for this service. At the time of writing, pharmacists are not recognized as health-care providers by the Centers for Medicare and Medicaid Services (CMS) and thus cannot be reimbursed directly by Medicare. Private insurance companies typically follow the standards set by Medicare, and thus may not cover pharmacist services either. The cost of a medication review by a pharmacist will vary based on the practice setting and payment model where the pharmacist works.

However, the federal government did give a nod to the value of medication reviews as a way to improve medication use and control costs. Namely, reviews are available at no charge to a subset of Medicare beneficiaries. With the launch in 2006 of the drug coverage portion of Medicare, all Part D drug plans are required to provide Medication Therapy Management (MTM) services to eligible beneficiaries. This program includes an annual medication review and is described in **Sidebar 3-2**.

SIDEBAR 3-2. MEDICARE PART D MEDICATION THERAPY MANAGEMENT SERVICES[84,85]

Medication Therapy Management (MTM) services were established in 2003 by the Medicare Modernization Act and further revised in 2010 under the Affordable Care Act. MTM services are a part of the Medicare Part D drug benefit and must be provided by Part D with the goal to reduce the risk of adverse drug events. There are two major components of the MTM requirement. One is a "targeted medication review" that focuses on a specific type of drug or medication-related problem. These reviews must occur on a quarterly basis and often involve identifying patients who can be switched to a less-expensive drug therapy option. The other component is a "comprehensive medication review" that involves a closer look at all of the medications that a beneficiary takes.

Comprehensive medication reviews must be offered to all "eligible" beneficiaries on an annual basis free of charge. However, who is "eligible" varies based on which Part D plan you are enrolled in. Each plan is allowed to set its own

Continued

specific criteria, as long as the following three conditions are met. The beneficiaries must: (1) have multiple health conditions; (2) use multiple medications; and (3) have a projected minimum annual drug expenditure as specified each year by the Center for Medicare and Medicaid Services (CMS). Each plan decides which specific health conditions a person must have and the number of medications a person must be prescribed to qualify. As a result, there is no national set of criteria.

Beneficiaries who are eligible are automatically enrolled in MTM services by their Part D plan and may opt out if they choose. MTM services, including comprehensive medication reviews, can be provided by a pharmacist or other "qualified provider." In addition, the services can be provided in-person, by telephone, or by telehealth, adding to the wide variability in how the comprehensive medication reviews are provided by Part D plans. Of note, not all plans utilize pharmacists to provide MTM services.

The concept of including a comprehensive review for selected older adults in Part D plans is a big step forward in recognizing the value of a complete medication review. However, only about 25 percent of eligible Medicare beneficiaries receive this comprehensive review.[86] Most beneficiaries simply are not aware of this service and may decline it, not realizing what is being offered to them. Thus, individuals may wish to contact their Part D plan to find out if they are eligible for a review at no charge.

SUMMARY

This chapter explains eight types of MRPs, along with efforts that you and your healthcare team can take to prevent them. Unfortunately, it is not possible to avoid all medication problems, but understanding the scope of

MRPs helps you to become a smarter consumer who is more engaged in how you take and manage your medications. Other chapters in this book provide greater detail about specific types of MRPs. The chapters in Part V focus on specific strategies that empower individuals to take a more active role to reduce the risk of MRPs. Important steps you can take include learning more about the medications you take, being more involved in medication decisions, and requesting a medication review once a year.

KEY POINTS

- A medication-related problem (MRP) is a potential or actual event regarding drug therapy that interferes with the ability to achieve a desired health outcome.
- Eight categories of medication-related problems have been defined and provide a framework for assessing a patient's drug therapy for preventable problems.
- The majority of medication-related problems can be prevented through careful prescribing and drug selection, drug therapy monitoring, and patient education.
- A comprehensive medication review is an important tool to identify and correct medication-related problems. It can improve health outcomes and reduce the risk of serious adverse events.

Part II

The Overmedication Problem

Chapter 4

Defining Polypharmacy

Ingrained in my memory is a lovely couple who asked me to review the husband's drug therapy. Anita and George were happily married and living in their home of many years where they had raised their children, now long grown and moved away. Anita was a devoted wife and actively involved in helping her husband manage his health and medications. As I joined them at their kitchen table, Anita waved a piece of paper at me. She explained it was a prescription for a new medication the doctor had prescribed for George. She waved her hand across the line of amber prescription bottles spread on the table and asked, "Why would he want to fill one more prescription? Look at all that he's already taking?" Anita and George's story has stayed with me all these years. It is a common fact that medication lists are growing longer, and patients too often struggle with a host of concerns and questions about their regimens. If you have ever felt like you take too many medications, you are not alone.

The word for using multiple medications is polypharmacy. "Poly" means many or multiple, and "pharmacy" refers to medications. Technically, polypharmacy implies neither something good nor bad. However, it has earned a bad reputation because taking multiple medications is one of the factors that increases the risk of experiencing a medication-related problem (MRP). From Anita and George's kitchen table to national think tanks, negative health outcomes that arise from excessive medication use no longer are being ignored. Polypharmacy has emerged as a national and global health concern, with a growing awareness of the particular risks to older individuals. I am aware of several notable events in recent years that illustrate how polypharmacy is seeping into our national conversation. Importantly, this conversation includes consumers as well as professionals and policymakers (see **Figure 4-1**).

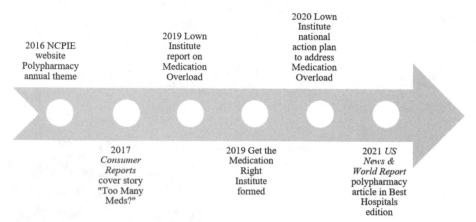

Figure 4-1. Timeline of Growing Awareness of Polypharmacy and Overmedication Use

The National Council on Patient Information and Education (NCPIE; now part of NeedyMeds) is a well-respected consumer advocacy organization that focuses on promoting responsible medication use to a consumer-based audience. In 2016, it chose polypharmacy as its annual theme, with a subtitle of "America's other drug problem."[87] The following year, the September cover story of *Consumer Reports* was "Too Many Meds?" further drawing consumers' attention to the problem of overmedication.[88] In 2019, the Lown Institute shifted the focus to the older adult population with its report, "Medication Overload, America's Other Drug Problem." The Lown Institute is a national nonpartisan think tank that advocates for healthcare reform. Using clear language and graphics, its report explains the causes and dangers of excessive medication use among older adults and highlights the impending clinical and economic impacts if we continue the status quo.[89] This initial report was followed by "Eliminating Medication Overload: A National Action Plan" in 2020. This second report makes specific recommendations to clinicians, healthcare organizations, government agencies, and patient advocacy groups about actions to counter the ongoing prescribing epidemic.[90]

At the same time these Lown reports were published, a new advocacy group called Get the Medications Right (GTMRx) Institute was created to assemble health-care professionals, organizations that pay for health care, consumer groups, and others with a shared interest in tackling the growing problem of excessive and costly inappropriate medication use. In its first three years, GTMRx grew to 1600 members. This group advocates for a patient-centered and team-based approach to improve medication use and ultimately improve health outcomes and reduce healthcare costs. A core principle of its approach is greater patient engagement in drug-therapy decisions.[91]

Finally, tucked inside the *US News and World Report's* "Best Hospitals 2021" edition was a two-page article highlighting polypharmacy in older adults.[92] The article, though succinct, references the Lown Institute reports and offers suggestions for how individuals together with their physicians can reduce medication use. This timeline of recent activity points toward a growing trend to make polypharmacy a household term. The time is now to talk about overuse of medications and put polypharmacy at the forefront of discussions among patients, prescribers, payers, and policy makers.

DIFFERENT WAYS TO DEFINE POLYPHARMACY

Polypharmacy in its most basic sense means the use of multiple medications. Use of prescription drugs is implied, but regular use of nonprescription medications certainly can be included in the count. There is no hard and fast rule. There also is no universally accepted definition of "multiple." The most common threshold is five or more medications,[93] but this number is arbitrary and can range from four to eleven, depending on the setting or researcher's preference. Using the common cutoff of five or more medications, polypharmacy is more than twice as common in older adults (42 percent) than in individuals age eighteen and older (around 20 percent).[94]

While the sheer number of medications a person takes can lead to negative health outcomes, this is not always the case. There are many situations where *appropriate* polypharmacy is warranted and helpful. With careful dosing, drug selection, and monitoring, the intent is that patients will benefit from drug therapy and experience few, if any, problems. Indeed, proper management of some of the most common health conditions in older adults requires two to four drugs, based on clinical guidelines. Examples of appropriate polypharmacy include the following:

- Hypertension (high blood pressure) often requires at least two medications to reach the goal of less than 130/80 mmHg.
- Diabetes often requires a combination of two or three drugs to control blood glucose levels plus the addition of a statin drug (common cholesterol medication) to manage heart-related (cardiovascular) risks.
- Patients who have had a heart attack or other evidence of coronary artery disease typically require a combination of three or more drugs: aspirin, a statin drug to lower cholesterol, plus medications to control blood pressure and prevent chest pain.
- Updated guidelines for the management of heart failure recommend a potential mix of at least four medications for most patients.

Thus, the number of medications alone can be of limited value when assessing if a person is taking too many medications. It also is necessary to look at which specific drugs a person is taking and the reason for each one. To this end, a more meaningful definition of polypharmacy is one that goes beyond simply a number.

This takes us to a second definition of polypharmacy: the use of medications that are not clinically needed or that are harmful or not effective.[95,96] This descriptive or qualitative definition captures the negative issues that surround excessive and *inappropriate* polypharmacy. Especially among the older population that is more susceptible to the negative or unwanted effects of medications, inappropriate polypharmacy clearly becomes something we strive to avoid. We can do this by removing harmful and unneeded drugs, lowering drug dosages, switching to safer medication options, and focusing on nondrug ways to manage a condition where possible.

You may be concerned as you read this chapter, knowing that you or your loved one takes five or more medications. Rest assured this does not mean that you are bound to have a medication-related problem or that your doctor has done something wrong. Appropriate polypharmacy exists. However, being attuned to the potential that medications have both wanted and unwanted effects places you in a more vigilant mindset. Regular medication reviews and discussions with your healthcare providers are warranted to evaluate drug therapy and prevent problems before they occur. **Sidebar 4-1** provides an example of a patient with polypharmacy to illustrate how we need to look more specifically at what is prescribed to fully assess whether appropriate or inappropriate polypharmacy is present.

MEDICATION OVERLOAD

Medication overload is another term for *inappropriate* polypharmacy. As mentioned earlier, the Lown Institute introduced this term with its report "Medication Overload: America's Other Drug Problem": "As the number of prescriptions has exploded, so has the frequency of polypharmacy-related harm, what we refer to … as medication overload."[97] The report states more specifically that medication overload is the use of multiple medications for which the risk of harm from a person's drug therapy is greater than the benefit.[98] The report summarizes the extent of the problem, harms that are related to medication overload, and factors that contribute to widespread overuse of medications.

The follow-up report, "Eliminating Medication Overload: A National Call to Action," provides specific recommendations to address the problem.[99] One of the recommendations is to create an awareness campaign about medication overload to educate patients, family members, and caregivers, as well as health professionals and policymakers. We need everyone who is impacted by medication overload to be fully aware of its scope and implications. Then and only then can we hope for meaningful change. Another recommendation is for clinicians to provide "prescription check-ups" that are focused specifically on relieving medication overload and stopping or reducing medications for patients who need it.[100] This requires a shift in mindset. Clinicians need to view prescribing with an eye toward stopping or reducing medications, rather than prescribing a medication that is destined to become a lifelong therapy.

The report concludes by recommending specific actions that patients and family members can take now to "begin the process of eliminating medication overload."[101] One action is to learn about the risks of excessive drug therapy. Another action is for patients and family members who have trouble managing medications or are worried about side effects to ask their physicians for a prescription checkup to identify opportunities to reduce overload. Both reports can be accessed online at the Lown Institute's website (https://lowninstitute.org/).

SIDEBAR 4-1. AN EXAMPLE OF POLYPHARMACY: APPROPRIATE OR INAPPROPRIATE?

Russ is seventy-two years old; he is retired but stays active with volunteer activities and social events. He lives on his own and has four grown children who live in town. This past year he has been focused on losing weight, exercising more regularly, and adopting healthier eating habits. He asked for a medication review because he feels like he is taking too many ("It's kind of overwhelming"), and his daughter finally convinced him a review will be helpful. He knows why some but not all of them are prescribed.

He has several health conditions for which he has regular check-ups with his primary care doctor and

cardiologist. He had a heart attack five years ago that was
treated with three-vessel bypass heart surgery. He has
high blood pressure, high cholesterol, gout, and arthritis
in his knees. Six months ago he was diagnosed with type
2 diabetes, which was part of his motivation to make
healthier lifestyle choices. His medication list is as follows.
Prescription medications:

1. Allopurinol 300 mg once daily
2. Amlodipine (Norvasc®) 10 mg once daily
3. Atorvastatin (Lipitor®) 40 mg once daily
4. Carvedilol (Coreg®) 25 mg twice daily
5. Isosorbide mononitrate (ISMN) ER (ImDur®) 30 mg
   once daily
6. Lisinopril (Prinivil®) 10 mg once daily
7. Empagliflozin (Jardiance®) 25 mg once daily
8. Zolpidem (Ambien®) 10 mg once daily at bedtime
9. Nitroglycerin 0.4 mg sublingual tablets, as needed for
   chest pain

Nonprescription medications:

1. Acetaminophen (Tylenol®) 500 mg three times daily
2. Aspirin 81 mg once daily
3. Fish oil supplement 1000 mg twice daily (dietary
   supplement)

Russ shared the following information with me during
the medication interview. He says the acetaminophen is
helpful for his knee pain. He started taking fish oil years
ago because his friend was taking it and said it was good
for the heart. He can't recall any episodes of chest pain

Continued

and has not used the nitroglycerin tablets "for years." His last gout attack was over two years ago. He has headaches sometimes after his morning medications and feels dizzy when he stands up too quickly. He said that he's had a couple stumbles ("It's my legs" he explained), and fell one time—at night on his way to the bathroom, but in general, he sleeps okay.

Russ is taking eleven medications on a regular basis; thus, based on a definition of five or more medications, he is experiencing polypharmacy. But is it appropriate polypharmacy or inappropriate polypharmacy and medication overload? To figure this out, each medication must be assessed in light of Russ's specific health situation.

Because Russ had a heart attack and bypass surgery, he has a diagnosis of coronary artery disease (CAD). Both aspirin and atorvastatin are appropriate medications in CAD to help prevent a second heart attack. Note that although aspirin is nonprescription, it is an important heart medication for Russ. His blood pressure needs to be well-controlled to prevent further heart disease and long-term health complications. He is prescribed amlodipine, carvedilol, and lisinopril, which all lower blood pressure plus have other heart benefits, including management of CAD. Benefits need to be weighed against risks, though. Some blood pressure medicines can cause or contribute to dizziness when Russ stands up too quickly. Also, it is likely that his weight loss and lifestyle changes have improved his blood pressure control since the medicines were first prescribed. Russ recalls that his doctor always says his blood pressure is doing really well. Taking three blood pressure medications at this point might be excessive for Russ and contribute to his dizziness upon standing.

Isosorbide mononitrate (ISMN) appears to be unnecessary and should be discussed with his physician. Russ has not had any episodes of chest pain in a long while, plus he's made positive changes to his eating and exercise habits that have improved management of his CAD. Notably, he is experiencing possible side effects of ISMN, namely dizziness and headache. Fish oil likely also is unnecessary. Russ started taking it on his own because of perceived heart benefits. While the trend years ago favored fish oil, more recently this has been questioned. In addition, it interacts with aspirin, and high doses increase the risk of bleeding.

Allopurinol for preventing gout flares generally is considered appropriate to continue. If it is stopped, a gout flare could occur again. However, if Russ has strong concerns about cost or side effects, and if his uric acid levels are within normal range, this medication could be considered for deprescribing based on person-centered care. Acetaminophen is a good choice for osteoarthritis pain and Russ says it is helpful, thus this drug is appropriate to continue. Empagliflozin is an appropriate medication for treating type 2 diabetes.

Last but definitely not least, zolpidem is a drug without an indication on Russ's list and is associated with important side effects in older adults. He does not have a diagnosis of chronic insomnia; plus, zolpidem can contribute to excessive sedation, falls, bone fracture, and motor vehicle accidents. It likely contributed to his "stumbles" and the fall he had. Experts recommend avoiding zolpidem in older adults. In light of the risk of harm and an unclear reason why this medication is prescribed, zolpidem is considered inappropriate polypharmacy and should be discussed with his physician.

Continued

In this case scenario, you can see how there are several unnecessary or possibly harmful medications that Russ is taking that are mixed in with important and beneficial drug therapy. It is important to understand that the need for certain medication can change over time as an individual's health changes and medical knowledge evolves. Russ's story illustrates the importance of routine reviews to tease out appropriate from inappropriate polypharmacy. As a rule, never stop or reduce a medication without first talking with your physician or pharmacist.

CAUSES OF POLYPHARMACY

How did we get to this state of widespread polypharmacy? It will be no surprise to learn that multiple contributing factors have been influencing medication use in the United States for years. Understanding the nature of these influences allows you to appreciate the breadth of the problem and be more prepared to stand up to these forces when feasible.

To begin with, as our population ages, there are more and more persons with multiple chronic conditions. Chronic health conditions go hand-in-hand with medication use. According to the Centers for Medicare and Medicaid Services (CMS), 69 percent of older adults are diagnosed with two or more chronic health conditions and 18 percent have six or more.[102] In contrast, just 27 percent of adults age eighteen and older report having more than one chronic health problem.[103] Health conditions common among older adults include high blood pressure, high cholesterol, arthritis, diabetes, and heart disease. The majority of these require drug therapy, and often more than one medication, as described earlier.

Another contributing factor is advances in medicine. As a result of improved medical knowledge, technology, and medications, we are able to survive health events that would have been devastating in the past, such as heart attacks, strokes, and cancer. Subsequently, we are living longer and have the opportunity to acquire other health conditions or ailments that call for drug therapy.

Polypharmacy also is driven by pharmaceutical advancements. Pharmaceutical science has allowed for an increasing number of drug discoveries. We now can treat medical conditions for which we had no drug therapy options in the past. Over the past three decades, the FDA approved an average of thirty-three novel new drugs per year.[104] That amounts to over a thousand new drugs during my career so far as a pharmacist. We also have seen a growth in the number of dietary supplements and over-the-counter (OTC) products on the market. These are multibillion dollar industries that heavily advertise to consumers.

Advertisements for prescription drugs contribute to polypharmacy trends as well. Since 1997, regulations in the United States have allowed pharmaceutical manufacturers to advertise prescription-only medications directly to consumers, a practice known as direct-to-consumer-advertising (DTCA). New Zealand is the only other country where this is legal. The impact of DTCA is complex and not without controversy. One of its benefits is increased awareness of certain health conditions that might be embarrassing for patients to talk about (such as overactive bladder or erectile dysfunction), which promotes physician-patient communication. On the other hand, DTCA is a lucrative opportunity, and drug companies spend about $6 billion annually in advertising to reach consumers. In a 2021 analysis, drugs with the highest DTCA spending were also noted to have the highest Medicare expenditures.[105]

Increased access to health information on the internet also has influenced widespread polypharmacy. As patients seek information about a health condition and its treatment options, they are more apt to self-treat with nonprescription medications or request a prescription from their physicians.

With the wide availability of prescription and nonprescription medications, coupled with high exposure through marketing and the internet, consumers are immersed in the message that pharmaceuticals will treat just about every ailment or symptom. This has contributed to a pill-popping culture, in which individuals tend to prefer a "pill for every ill." It is far easier to swallow a medication than to invest time and effort in life-style changes and other nondrug treatments. Unfortunately, patients often expect a prescription from their physicians when they describe a symptom, and many times physicians will oblige because they are trained to be healers and want to address their patients' needs. I have heard many stories from patients who were prescribed a medication to treat a symptom because the patient happened to mention it at the doctor's office. For example, "I told my doctor my stomach was bothering me" or "I said I felt nervous sometimes," and the patient was handed another prescription, when quite possibly watching, waiting, or discussing options would have been effective. The term "slow medicine" captures the concept of taking time to pause, consider the whole patient, and discuss with the individual both benefits and harms of various treatment options.[106] The phrase contrasts with the typical fast-pace of medicine that is marked by intervening with procedures and prescriptions that may or may not be helpful.

Physicians also contribute to polypharmacy trends, with several factors at play. Many doctors lack geriatric training and therefore have less knowledge of polypharmacy issues. In turn, they might prescribe more freely a new medication rather than evaluate other options. Another factor is that physicians often are hesitant to adjust or stop medications that were initially prescribed by someone else; thus, medications can be continued unnecessarily.[107] Time constraints during office appointments play a role and are driven at least in part by insurance reimbursement policies. Limited time with patients means that physicians are hard-pressed to confirm and review an accurate medication list, listen to the person's goals and preferences, and discuss options—drug or non-drug—before deciding whether a new prescription is appropriate. Finally, physicians also must navigate payment policies that create incentives to prescribe medications according to the latest clinical practice guidelines. Practice guidelines set the gold standard for treatment of individual health conditions. However, they rarely take into consideration older patients who have multiple health conditions. As a result, when different clinical practice guidelines are applied to one individual, it can lead to excessive prescribing and a complex regimen that does more harm than good.[108,109]

A final contributing factor to polypharmacy is increased affordability of and access to medications because of insurance coverage. In 2006, medication insurance was made available to older adults enrolled in Medicare through the newly established Medicare Part D program. Medication utilization among Medicare beneficiaries increased in that first year by about 6 percent.[110] Since that time, Medicare Part D plans have continued to evolve, as have Medicare Advantage plans that also offer prescription drug coverage.

DEPRESCRIBING

I have heard more than once from my clients, "My doctors are quick to add a new medication, but they've never stopped any of them." The idea of stopping drug therapy is not new, but there is a relatively new term for it: deprescribing. Deprescribing is the systematic process of reducing dosages or stopping medications that no longer are needed or no longer benefit the patient. The process involves not only discontinuing (stopping) a drug, but also adjusting therapy by switching to a safer choice or reducing a dosage when needed.[111] Research that provides more evidence on when and how to deprescribe medicines safely is expanding rapidly and reflects growing interest in this topic.

Safe and appropriate medication use ideally should include plans to stop a medication when it no longer is needed or effective, or if it is causing side effects. Most medications are not meant to be taken forever. Unfortunately, in current clinical practice, we do not routinely seek out ways to reduce drug therapy. And thus, medication lists continue to grow. When patients bring up a new symptom, physicians are trained to help by "doing something," and the quickest and easiest thing often is to write a new prescription.

Stopping drug therapy is not as easy as it sounds. There are numerous barriers to overcome. Research consistently shows that three out of four individuals want to reduce the number of medications they take, and more than 90 percent indicate they are willing to stop medicines if their physician says it is possible. However, actual deprescribing occurs infrequently.[112,113,114] Patients can become hesitant for various reasons. They might be fearful that symptoms will return or their health condition will worsen. They do not want to upset their doctors by bringing up the question of stopping medications. Many individuals grow accustomed to taking their medications and are reluctant to let go of a comfortable routine. Finally, if their doctor brings up stopping a medicine, patients might think the doctor is giving up or abandoning them and thus view deprescribing as a bad thing.[115,116]

Physicians experience barriers to deprescribing, too. Physicians widely agree that they lack sufficient knowledge and guidance. How to stop drugs is not included in basic medical school curriculum. Clinical practice guidelines provide information on when to add medications, but fail to address when they might be stopped. As a result, clinicians are left without guidance on how to reduce or remove medications once prescribed. Another barrier is that physicians do not want to change a medication prescribed by one of their colleagues. Additionally, information often is lacking in a patient's health record about why a drug was started years ago, making it difficult for someone to determine if deprescribing is appropriate. Finally, efforts to discontinue a medication require extra time and follow-up that often is just not available in the current structure and payment model of our health-care system.[117,118] Unless there is an overt problem, it is easiest to renew prescriptions and continue the same medication list. We call this prescribing inertia.

Deprescribing is possible but it requires a very person-centered approach, as everyone's situation is unique. Success is achieved when clinicians work with one patient at a time to reduce unnecessary or harmful medications and address other drug therapy problems. Ultimately, greater patient engagement is a key component to being able to reduce or stop medications. However, many individuals are not even aware that deprescribing is an option. Clearly, greater awareness is needed. Research on deprescribing continues to grow and evolve. In turn, more resources eventually will become available to help guide clinicians and patients when making decisions to stop, reduce, or continue drug therapy.

SUMMARY

As our nation continues to age, we have in the United States a prescribing epidemic that demands our attention. The growing presence of excessive medication use is a major concern for older adults and public health in general. Medications are vital for managing chronic conditions and to improve our well-being. However, problems can arise when we use medications without weighing benefits and harms or when there is a lack of coordination of care between prescribers. Fortunately, interest is gaining momentum at the national level to grow public awareness and engage healthcare professionals to take action to address the problem of inappropriate polypharmacy.

Deprescribing refers to stopping or reducing unnecessary medications. The process of deprescribing is an important tool to help tackle the medication overload problem. Research in this area is rapidly expanding to guide patients and clinicians on how to safely deprescribe medications. The next chapter continues this urgent conversation and addresses consequences of polypharmacy.

KEY POINTS

- Polypharmacy can be defined as the use of five or more medications, or more qualitatively as the use of medications that are unnecessary, ineffective, or harmful.
- Medication overload is defined as the use of multiple medications for which risk of harm from one's drug therapy is greater than the benefit.
- There are multiple factors that promote polypharmacy, including medical advances, increased availability of medications, patient and physician expectations, pharmaceutical advertisement to consumers, and cultural influences.
- Deprescribing refers to a systematic process to reduce unnecessary medications. Research is ongoing to better inform clinicians and patients about the safest ways to stop drug therapy.

Chapter 5

Consequences of Polypharmacy

Polypharmacy refers to taking multiple medications, commonly defined as five or more. Sometimes taking multiple medications is a good thing, and sometimes it can lead to trouble. Thus, we further define polypharmacy as being appropriate or inappropriate, as discussed in the previous chapter. Appropriate polypharmacy means that each drug has a valid medical reason for use and it is is judiciously prescribed and monitored. In this way, clinical benefits of drug therapy—appropriate use of polypharmacy—clearly outweigh potential harms. Appropriate polypharmacy is beneficial and improves one's health and well-being.

On the other hand, drug therapy that is inappropriate—that is not needed, harmful or ineffective—simply adds to the risk of possible harm without providing meaningful health benefits. It is this aspect of polypharmacy that burdens patients and our health system and contributes to the consequences summarized in this chapter.

It is hoped that a greater awareness of the potential harm of polypharmacy will help us feel more empowered and motivated to take actions individually and collectively to stem the tide of excessive medication use. Some general steps older adults and their family members can take to address polypharmacy are also provided, but more detailed recommendations are found in later chapters.

ADVERSE DRUG REACTIONS

One of the most common consequences of polypharmacy is an increased risk of adverse drug reactions (ADRs). ADRs are the unintended or unwanted effects of drugs. A more commonly used term is drug side effects, which is roughly interchangeable. Most of us are familiar with stories about a bad experience with a medication. Statistically, the chance of experiencing an ADR increases with the number of medications the person takes.[119] Of particular concern, older adults are three times more likely to have to go to an emergency department because of an adverse reaction compared to adults younger than sixty-five, and seven times more likely to be hospitalized.[120]

ADRs often are harder to detect in patients with polypharmacy. They are thus more likely to go unrecognized and can lead to what is called a "prescribing cascade." A prescribing cascade occurs when an ADR is incorrectly thought to be a new health problem, which then leads to another drug being prescribed to manage this "new" health condition, as depicted in **Figure 5-1**. A word of wisdom in geriatric care is to first assume a new symptom is a drug side effect, rather than jumping to the conclusion that it is a new ailment. For example, the dementia medication donepezil can increase urinary incontinence (decreased ability to hold urine), leading to more frequent urination. In turn, the physician might prescribe a drug to treat an overactive bladder, rather than recognize a possible side effect of donepezil. Instead of adding another drug, it might be more helpful to reassess the benefits and risks of donepezil in light of the new adverse reaction.

Susan's story illustrates another common prescribing cascade. When I met with her, her medication list included enalapril for treating blood pressure and dextromethorphan/guaifenesin to treat a chronic dry cough. The cough syrup caught my eye because it is unusual for someone to take it long-term. When I asked Susan, she explained that she had a dry cough that wouldn't go away. Her doctor suggested she try an over-the-counter cough medicine. As it turns out, the cough was due to enalapril, which has a side effect of a dry cough. Rather than add a cough medicine, her physician should have recognized the side effect and switched to a different

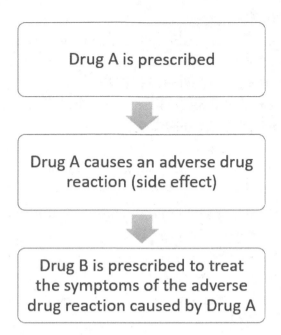

Figure 5-1. Prescribing Cascade

medicine for her blood pressure. Instead, the cough was seen as a new condition that needed another drug.

Another common example of a prescribing cascade occurs with the blood pressure medicine amlodipine. In higher doses, it can cause ankle swelling that is misdiagnosed as a new medical problem. In turn, patients frequently are prescribed a strong diuretic (water pill) such as furosemide to treat the fluid retention.[121]

A final note about ADRs and polypharmacy is that an ADR can appear as a vague symptom not clearly related to any one medication. For example, older individuals might experience dizziness, drowsiness, decreased appetite, or decreased memory. These symptoms can be mistaken as part of "normal" aging. In reality, none of these symptoms are normal; however, clinicians and patients alike can fall prey to stereotypes of ageism. Many times, patients might not bother to share these symptoms with their physicians. The result is that these types of less specific ADRs can be brushed off in error.[122]

DRUG INTERACTIONS

Drug interactions are a second important consequence of polypharmacy. The more medications a person takes, the greater the likelihood of having a clinically significant interaction. Medications can interact with another medication or with a health condition, food, alcohol, or marijuana. Non-prescription drugs like over-the-counter medications and dietary supplements also can interact with prescription drugs, as will be discussed in Chapter 6. Finally, interactions between drugs and health conditions (also known as disease states) are particularly important in older adults who frequently are diagnosed with multiple chronic conditions.

Many interactions are of a less serious nature and do not require an intervention. However, some interactions can be serious enough to necessitate an emergency department visit or hospitalization. Fortunately, most serious drug-drug interactions are well-documented and preventable in older adults.[123,124] Sufficient knowledge and proper monitoring are key. More detail about drug interactions, including examples of the different types, are found in Chapter 9.

MEDICATION ADHERENCE

Polypharmacy is associated with reduced medication adherence. This term (formerly called medication compliance) is defined as the extent to which a person correctly follows medication instructions. Adherence is an important topic that is more fully addressed in its own chapter. Poor medication adherence is common in older adults for a number of varied reasons. Longer medication lists typically involve more complex schedules for taking one's medications. Individuals can feel overwhelmed when they have to remember to take multiple pills every day and at different times, with some pills having special instructions to be taken with or without food, for example. A complex medication schedule is just one example of how polypharmacy can negatively impact adherence. Myriad other barriers can interfere with medication adherence and are discussed in Chapter 8. The downstream impact of poor adherence (not taking medications properly) is that a person's health conditions will go untreated or be poorly managed, leading to worsening health and progression of the condition. Tips and strategies to help improve adherence are provided in Chapter 17.

COGNITIVE AND PHYSICAL FUNCTION

Polypharmacy has been associated with impaired cognition, delirium (fluctuating changes in mental status), and dementia.[125,126,127] Physical function also can be negatively impacted. Studies have found an association between polypharmacy and increased falls, slower walking speed, decreased balance, and decreased grip strength.[128,129,130] Indeed, polypharmacy contributes to increased fall risk as a result of additive side effects such as dizziness, low blood pressure, and effects on balance.[131,132]

Annette is a seventy-eight-year-old woman who shared the following story with me that illustrates this point perfectly. She had fallen a few times and was concerned, of course. At her next office visit, she mentioned this to her physician. The doctor noted her blood pressure was running low, which could contribute to her falls. Annette said she also had improved her eating habits since her last doctor visit. This, too, can improve blood pressure, leading to a reduced need for medications. Her doctor ended up stopping two of Annette's blood pressure medicines, which corrected the problem.

HEALTH-CARE COSTS

Patients with polypharmacy have to deal with the direct costs or copays of every medication. For many older adults, the additive costs of their medications can become quite burdensome and contribute to poor adherence. It is not uncommon that patients have to choose between medications and groceries or other household expenses. Other costs associated with polypharmacy include those associated with monitoring drug therapy, such as costs of laboratory tests or the purchase of home monitoring supplies like a blood glucose monitor and test strips.

Government and private insurance companies also experience the financial burden of polypharmacy because it is associated with the increased use of health-care services such as additional outpatient visits, emergency department visits, and hospitalization.[133] In 2018, health-care costs from increased outpatient visits and hospitalizations due to ADRs and serious interactions were estimated to reach $3.8 billion.[134]

QUALITY OF LIFE

Finally, polypharmacy can have a negative impact on one's quality of life.[135] For some individuals, keeping track of multiple medications is an added mental stress. Patients have to manage multiple prescriptions and refills, know when and how to take them, and know why they are prescribed. Anxiety can increase because of concern about costs or fear of side effects.[136] Still other individuals tolerate vague or mild side effects, sometimes unaware they are symptoms caused by one or more of their medications. I've seen people miss out on activities outside of the house because they have side effects—for example, they feel too tired or they take a diuretic (water pill) and are fearful of not being able to get to a bathroom in time.

Polypharmacy is associated with a high pill burden—the total number of individual pills that a person has to take every day—that can have a negative impact on quality of life. I recall a patient who managed her pill burden by separating her pills so that she took just two or three at a time every three hours. She was content with her solution; yet it no doubt created another type of hassle for her.

Finally, older individuals eventually might need additional help to manage complex medicine regimens. This can create further stress and impact one's quality of life. I have spoken with many adult children who struggle because their parents want to remain in their own homes yet they are not able to manage their medications safely on their own. In far too many situations, difficulty self-managing medications at home is the reason an individual has to move to an assisted living facility or a nursing home.

PATIENT ROLE IN ADDRESSING POLYPHARMACY

Knowledge of the consequences of polypharmacy drives home the need to take only medications that are of benefit to our health. Remember that the use of nonprescription products contributes to polypharmacy, and these types of medications also need to be carefully considered. Ideally, patients need to learn about risks of medication overload and seek a prescription checkup specifically to reduce the number of medications. This is especially important when patients are troubled by side-effect concerns or have difficulty managing them.[137]

Talk with your healthcare team about polypharmacy and deprescribing. Knowledge of what these terms mean hopefully empowers you to be more confident to bring up these important topics. Studies show that patients who initiate the conversation with their physicians about their medications are more likely to be able reduce or stop them.[138] If you want to avoid unnecessary medications, say so! Advocating for yourself is key.

In the same breath, have confidence in the value of beneficial drug therapy to manage long-term conditions. In many instances, there might be nondrug strategies that can help you reduce the reliance on medications, but you need to discuss this with your physician. Do not neglect taking your essential medications every day. Make sure you have the tools to help you remember to take them and the support of family and friends to assist you with managing your medicines when needed.

An important word of caution is that you should never stop or make changes to a medication on your own without consulting your physician or pharmacist. Abruptly stopping certain medications can be dangerous and lead to withdrawal symptoms or a rebound of your health condition. If your physician and you agree to stop a medication, develop a plan for how to do it safely. Often a slow decrease of the dose is warranted. Ask about symptoms you can watch for, either withdrawal symptoms as the medication is reduced or stopped, or symptoms that signal a worsening or return of the health condition the drug was treating. Importantly, know what steps to take if symptoms occur. More information along with tips and strategies to address many of these recommendations are found in other chapters in this book.

SUMMARY

Medications can be of great benefit when they are used for a valid clinical reason and with ongoing monitoring for safety. However, polypharmacy or use of multiple medications can be associated with various consequences, ranging from increased risk of adverse drug reactions to reduced quality of life. Knowledge of these potential consequences helps us refocus on the importance of avoiding unnecessary medications. Additionally, it bolsters the argument that polypharmacy and associated consequences need to become part of mainstream conversations. National momentum must continue to engage patients, health-care professionals, and payers of health care to take action to reduce medication overload and inappropriate polypharmacy. Meanwhile, patients can work with their pharmacist and others on the health-care team to ensure they are taking their medications in a safe and effective manner to maximize benefit and reduce harm.

KEY POINTS

- Consequences of polypharmacy are multifold and include increased risk of adverse drug reactions and interactions, poor adherence, decreased cognitive and physical function, increased costs, and reduced quality of life.
- Medications that are truly helpful have health benefits that outweigh potential harms; careful prescribing and monitoring can limit the negative consequences.
- Patients need to be empowered to bring up the important topics of polypharmacy and deprescribing with their health-care professionals.
- Patients can help reduce medication overload by becoming more engaged in their health care and medication decisions and by asking their physicians about ways to reduce or stop medications.

Part III

Beyond Prescription Drugs

Chapter 6

Nonprescription Medications: Over-the-Counter Drugs and Dietary Supplements

Prescription drugs may get the headlines when we discuss safe and appropriate medication use, but drugs that are available without a prescription are just as important. There are two categories of nonprescription medications that are the subject of this chapter: over-the-counter (OTC) drugs and dietary supplements. People can access and use these drugs without ever interacting with a physician, pharmacist, or nurse, which makes them at once readily available to the public, but in the same breath this contributes to polypharmacy and an increased risk of medication-related problems (MRPs). Characteristics that make older adults more vulnerable to MRPs described in Chapter 2 apply to all medications, including OTC drugs and dietary supplements; adverse effects and interactions occur with these medications, too. Two additional categories of drugs are available without a prescription in the United States but are less commonly used and will not be addressed in this chapter; namely, homeopathic products and medical foods. Older adults might come across these types of products, thus a brief explanation of these categories is provided in **Sidebar 6-1.**

In my experience, older adults do not always view nonprescription products as "real" medications. Many people tend to overestimate safety of these products and believe that because they were purchased without a prescription, they do not need to be included on a medication list. When I ask clients to gather all of their medications for a medication review, they typically bring just their prescriptions. It is not uncommon that I have to remind people to show me *all* of the medications they take, even those not prescribed by their doctor. Even then, I often need to further remind clients to include things like aspirin, vitamins, and sleep aids.

Use of OTC drugs and dietary supplements is integral in our healthcare delivery system and an essential part of self-care choices. The term self-care refers to actions that individuals take to prevent disease, treat minor ailments, and manage chronic health conditions. Self-care can be broken down into two categories. One is self-care with nonprescription products like OTC drugs and dietary supplements, which is the focus of this chapter. The second is self-care that involves lifestyle choices and other nondrug strategies, which is the focus of the next chapter. Both aspects of self-care are essential to healthy aging.

Up to 40 percent of older adults do not use their OTC products appropriately.[139] While older individuals express that they are aware of and want to avoid adverse effects of nonprescription products, research also indicates they do not necessarily know which products are associated with greater risk.[140] At the national level, it is recognized that older adults need more education and information to empower them to use nonprescription medications safely and effectively.[141] Thus, this chapter focuses on these "other" drug categories. It will explain their risk and benefits and how they fit into the bigger scheme of safe medication use.

SIDEBAR 6-1. HOMEOPATHIC DRUGS AND MEDICAL FOODS

Homeopathic drugs are regulated as drugs by the FDA; however, they fall under a different set of regulations than prescription and OTC drugs. Homeopathic manufacturers are guided by the *US Homeopathic Pharmacopoeia*, which is the official listing of all homeopathic substances. Homeopathy is a form of complementary and alternative medicine (CAM). It is based on the principle that "like cures like," namely, if a substance can cause symptoms of an illness in large doses, it can provide a cure when given in very small doses. With homeopathic drugs, the more dilute the product is, the more potent it is thought to be. As a result, many homeopathic products contain little to no active ingredient and pose low risk of harm. However, they are not risk free. Some products have been found to contain measurable amounts of active drug ingredients or toxic contaminants that can harm individuals. Other concerns include improper manufacturing procedures and incorrect dilutions.

There currently are no FDA-approved homeopathic products on the market. Thus, any products being sold as homeopathic have not undergone FDA review to evaluate safety or effectiveness. Since 1988, homeopathic products have been marketed with the expectation that they follow the standards put forth in the Homeopathic Pharmacopoeia. In response to safety concerns, however, the FDA recently has shifted its approach to these products. In 2019, the FDA withdrew its long-standing policy for homeopathic remedies in favor of stricter oversight. At the time of writing, new regulations have not yet been finalized, but closer regulation of homeopathic products is anticipated.

Medical foods are foods designed for specific dietary management of diseases that have distinctive nutritional requirements. They technically can be accessed without a prescription; however, medical foods are intended for use only under medical supervision and thus often are prescribed

Continued

to patients. In contrast to homeopathic products, medical foods are not regulated as drugs. They are differentiated from the broader category of foods because they must be specifically formulated for use in meeting a nutritional requirement for a disease or condition. They cannot be naturally occurring foods or foods that a physician might recommend as part of an overall diet. The first medical foods were developed to treat inborn errors of metabolism, such as phenylketonuria (PKU). In recent years, medical foods have been marketed for conditions seen in older adults, such as nerve pain and dementia, among others. Medical foods are considered generally safe and effective by the FDA. Manufacturers of medical foods must abide by regulations for labeling and good manufacturing processes.

TERMINOLOGY

In this book, I will use "nonprescription" as an umbrella term that encompasses both OTC products and dietary supplements. Each of these more specific categories is described in detail below. Neither category requires a physician's order (that is, a prescription) to purchase or access these medicines. As such, I have chosen to group them together as nonprescription products. However, this is a little unconventional and is where their similarities end, as discussed in the next section. In other publications and resources, the term "nonprescription" more commonly refers only to OTC drugs and not dietary supplements.

Another liberty I take in this chapter and throughout the book is to refer to dietary supplements as medications or drugs. From a regulatory standpoint they are not drugs, as will be explained. However, it is of paramount importance to recognize that dietary supplements have pharmacologic activity in the body; they can contribute to adverse effects and drug interactions, and the rules of pharmacokinetics and pharmacodynamics still apply. Thus, from a safety standpoint, it makes sense to view supplements along the same lines as OTC and prescribed medications.

OVERVIEW OF NONPRESCRIPTION PRODUCTS

The OTC and dietary supplement markets continue to grow year after year. Consumers spend more than $40 billion annually on these products.[142] The Food and Drug Administration (FDA) estimates that there are about 300,000 OTC products[143] and 80,000 dietary supplements from which consumers can choose.[144] Common OTC products include antacids, cough and cold products, laxatives, and pain relievers such as acetaminophen, ibuprofen, and naproxen. Not to be overlooked, aspirin is an OTC product that is widely used as part of a prescribed regimen to reduce heart attack and stroke risk. Examples of common dietary supplements include vitamins, calcium, and fish oil; others are listed in **Table 6-1**.

Table 6-1. Examples of Common Dietary Supplements

Type of supplement	Examples
Vitamins	Multivitamin combinations Vitamin B_{12} Vitamin D_3
Minerals	Calcium Iron Magnesium
Herbals	Gingko biloba St. John's wort Turmeric
Amino acids and other naturally-derived products	Glucosamine and chondroitin Melatonin Omega-3 fatty acids, fish oil

Nonprescription products can be purchased at retail stores ranging from supermarkets to gas stations and are a click away on the internet. They offer individuals independence in managing minor ailments, as well as easy access. Ideally, use of nonprescription products as part of self-care treatment is a way to reduce health-care costs. Not only are the products less expensive than prescribed medications, but when used properly, they can prevent bigger health issues from developing. Indeed, many nonprescription products are relied on for treatment of health conditions common to older adults. For example, management of heartburn and reflux symptoms calls for use of antacids, histamine$_2$-receptor blockers (such as famotidine), and proton pump inhibitors (such as omeprazole). Treatment of osteoporosis includes adequate intake of calcium and vitamin D along with prescribed medications. Patients who are deficient in vitamin D or iron might be instructed by their physician to take a vitamin D or iron supplement to replace low levels.

PREVALENCE OF USE

Use of nonprescription products is widespread, with older adults being among the biggest consumers. Nearly 40 percent of older adults use OTC products and more than 70 percent use dietary supplements.[145,146] More than one-half of older adults take multiple dietary supplements.[147] Furthermore, these products commonly are combined with prescription medications. Yet, most people do not tell their physicians about nonprescription products they use.[148] A study published in the *Journal of the American Medical Association* estimated that 15 percent of older adults are at risk of experiencing a major drug interaction between prescription and nonprescription drugs.[149]

REGULATION

To most consumers, the categories of OTC drugs and dietary supplements blend together. Separating them into two groups may not make sense on the surface. However, critical differences exist, beginning with how they are defined and regulated, which ultimately impact how to safely approach the use of each category. These differences are discussed next and summarized in **Table 6-2.**

Table 6-2. Regulation of Over-the-Counter (OTC) Products and Dietary Supplements

	OTC Products	Dietary Supplements
Regulating body	FDA	FDA
Product category	Drug	Food
Evidence of safety and effectiveness	Manufacturer must prove safety and effectiveness before marketing or market a product that is made up of accepted OTC ingredients (as defined by the OTC monographs).	Manufacturer is not required to provide evidence of safety or effectiveness; burden lies with FDA to prove a product is unsafe or mislabeled only after it is marketed.
Manufacturing standards	Purity and quality must meet same high standards as for prescription drug manufacturing. OTC manufacturers are required to adhere to current Good Manufacturing Practices.	Purity and quality unknown; manufacturers are encouraged to follow Good Manufacturing Practices but manufacturers are responsible for ensuring their products meet FDA regulations. FDA can take action only after a product is marketed.

OTC products are regulated as *drugs* by the FDA in the same strict manner as are prescription drugs. A drug is defined by the FDA as a substance intended to diagnose, cure, mitigate, treat, or prevent disease. The definition further states that drugs are intended "to affect the structure or any function of the body."[150] Thus, labels of OTC products are permitted to state what the product treats, for example, "effective relief of constipation" or "prevents and relieves heartburn."

Regulation of drugs as we know them today—both prescription and OTC products—has been evolving for nearly a hundred years and continues to undergo modifications. Of notable historic interest, it was not until 1962 that the government required that drugs must be proven effective in addition to being safe as a prerequisite for FDA approval.[151] As a result, new prescription drugs today by and large have undergone rigorous clinical studies to prove safety and effectiveness before reaching the consumer. The OTC drug category was created in 1951 with the passage of a law that established prescription-only status for certain medications, leaving the remaining drugs to become what we know of today as OTC products.[152]

Currently, there are two common regulatory pathways by which a drug can be approved for OTC use. The first pathway is called the OTC monograph pathway, which began in 1972 when the FDA initiated a massive OTC Drug Review process to confirm the safety and effectiveness of all OTC active ingredients.[153] As part of the monograph pathway, the FDA grouped all existing OTC ingredients into therapeutic categories (such as laxatives or antacids, for example) and created a drug monograph for each category. The drug monographs define ingredients that are deemed acceptable for use in OTC products, and together the monographs make up a "rule book" for drug manufacturers. In this way, manufacturers can market OTC products without needing specific approval by the FDA, as long as they follow the rules laid out in the monographs. The majority of our current OTC products are available via this pathway.

The other common route for approval of an OTC product is to transition from prescription to OTC status. Since 1976, over a hundred drugs have been reclassified in this way (see **Table 6-3**).[154] Prescription-to-OTC products have undergone the rigorous safety and effectiveness testing that is required of prescription drugs, and thus have a more assured effectiveness profile compared to products from the monograph pathway. The drawn-out OTC Review Process has not yet been completed. Thus, in 2020, legislation was passed to modernize the OTC Review Process and allow the FDA to more quickly respond to safety concerns with OTC products.[155]

Table 6-3. Examples of Prescription-to-OTC-Switches

Drug class	Generic name (brand name)	Year switched to OTC
Proton pump inhibitors	Omeprazole (Prilosec®)	2003
	Lansoprazole (Prevacid®)	2009
	Esomeprazole (Nexium®)	2014
Allergy medications	Fluticasone nasal spray (Flonase®)	2014
	Budesonide nasal spray (Rhinocort®)	2015
	Olopatadine eye drops (Pataday®)	2020
	Azelastine nasal spray (Astepro®)	2021
Topical pain medication	Diclofenac sodium topical gel (Voltaren® Gel)	2020

Dietary supplements are regulated as *foods* by the FDA. The major law that affects the current status of dietary supplements was passed in 1994 and is called the Dietary Supplement Health and Education Act (DSHEA). DSHEA defines a dietary supplement as a product that contains an herbal product, mineral, vitamin, or amino acid that is taken by mouth and intended to supplement the diet.[156] By law, dietary supplement labeling cannot make any therapeutic or health claims, in contrast to OTC products. The manufacturer instead is limited to "structure and function" claims of how the dietary supplement affects the human body. To illustrate this, a calcium supplement can state that it builds strong bones but cannot state that it treats osteoporosis. Other acceptable statements include "supports bone, teeth, and muscle health" and "helps support a healthy heart, brain, and eyes." Any time a structure and function claim is made, it must be accompanied by a disclaimer that states that the claim has not been evaluated by the FDA and that the product "is not intended to diagnose, treat, cure, or prevent any disease."

As a result of DSHEA, the FDA has far less ability to regulate dietary supplements compared to the oversight it has for drug products, and the oversight happens only after a supplement is made available to the public. Manufacturers of dietary supplements have the responsibility to make sure their products are safe and that labeling meets federal requirements. However, safety data do not have to be submitted to the government and labeling does not have to be pre-approved. In fact, the manufacturer has thirty days after the product is marketed to submit a copy of the label to the FDA, leaving the federal agency with the burden to react to safety concerns or noncompliance only after a product is on retail shelves.[157] This is in stark contrast to the emphasis on premarketing documentation required for drug products. There is no requirement for supplement manufacturers to submit information on effectiveness, dosage, interactions, or adverse effects. No studies are required for specific age groups such as children or older adults. In short, the bar is set much lower for safety and effectiveness requirements for dietary supplements. The mantra "buyer beware" rings true.

Clearly, these several differences between OTC drugs and dietary supplements in the eyes of the FDA are important because they have direct implications for consumers. FDA regulation of OTC drugs provides a high level of comfort that these products by and large are effective and safe when instructions for use are followed. For dietary supplements, however, consumers need to be aware that there are no requirements for safety and effectiveness. The burden of proof falls on the FDA to show that a dietary supplement is unsafe and needs to be withdrawn from the market. In response to safety concerns, DSHEA was amended in 2007 to improve manufacturing safety, and subsequent regulations boosted the requirements for makers of dietary supplements to report serious adverse events.[158,159] However, the fact remains that oversight of the supplement industry is reactive rather than proactive.

SAFE AND EFFECTIVE USE OF NONPRESCRIPTION PRODUCTS

OTC drugs and dietary supplements have the potential to cause or contribute to MRPs in older adults, thus individuals need to weigh the benefits against possible harms before taking any of these products. Safe selection and use of nonprescription products by older individuals can be more complicated because of the presence of multiple chronic conditions and prescribed medications. In addition, older adults experience age-related physiologic changes, namely pharmacokinetic and pharmacodynamic changes as explained in Chapter 2. Importantly, the health-care team needs to be informed of any nonprescription products that a patient takes. Having a medication list that includes an individual's nonprescription products is essential whenever medications are reviewed. Unfortunately, there are too many reports of patients who experience a preventable adverse effect that involves an OTC or supplement that the physician or pharmacist did not know the patient was taking.

As explained earlier, drugs that fall into the OTC category are deemed to have a fairly large window of safety. With appropriate labeling, consumers should be able to properly use these drugs without medical supervision. However, certain OTC products need to be approached with greater caution in older adults because they are associated with an increased risk of adverse effects as highlighted in **Table 6-4**. In some situations, when significant risk factors are present, they should be avoided altogether.

Table 6-4. Over-the-Counter Products Associated with an Increased Risk of Adverse Effects in Older Adults

Drug/drug class	Common brand names	Adverse drug reaction risk
Acetaminophen	Tylenol®	Liver toxicity, especially if combined with alcohol
Antihistamines, first generation: diphenhydramine, chlorpheniramine, doxylamine	Benadryl®, Coricidin®, Advil® PM, Tylenol® PM, Unisom®, others	Decreased memory, confusion, dry eyes, dry mouth, blurred vision, constipation
Aspirin	Bayer®, Bufferin®, St. Joseph®, others	Bleeding risk
Nonsteroidal anti-inflammatory drugs (NSAIDs): ibuprofen, naproxen	Advil®, Aleve®	Stomach ulcers, bleeding risk, kidney problems, risk of stroke or heart attack; increased blood pressure

OTC drugs have several well-known interactions with prescription drugs and health conditions. For example, aspirin and nonsteroidal anti-inflammatory drugs (NSAIDs) increase the risk of bleeding when combined with prescription medications that reduce blood clots (anticoagulant or antiplatelet agents). NSAIDs can increase blood pressure and worsen heart failure symptoms. Many antihistamines and decongestants—common components of cough and cold products—can worsen symptoms of an enlarged prostate. Acetaminophen (the generic drug in Tylenol®) is a concern because of the potential to ingest more than is safe as a result of acetaminophen being found in multiple products. This risk is discussed in more detail later in this chapter.

Some OTC ingredients are of questionable effectiveness but remain on the market. Examples include the decongestant phenylephrine, cough medicines guaifenesin and dextromethorphan, and antihistamines when used alone to treat symptoms of the common cold.[160,161] As an aside, these products of questionable effectiveness were approved via the older monograph process, rather than the more rigorous prescription-to-OTC process. Checking with a pharmacist or physician can guide individuals toward more beneficial ingredients and effective nondrug options.

Dietary supplements have a separate set of considerations for safe and effective use. The major concern with these products is that clinical studies to support safety and effectiveness are not required. Consequently, there usually is very limited information available about how the supplement works in the body, what is an appropriate dose, and if there are any significant interactions or side effects. Information on safe use in older adults typically is even rarer. There are several well-known interactions with dietary supplements, and examples of these are provided in **Table 6-5**.

Table 6-5. Examples of Significant Drug Interactions with Dietary Supplements

Dietary supplements	Interacting drugs	Potential adverse effect
Garlic, Ginseng, Gingko biloba Vitamin E	Anticoagulants (warfarin, apixaban, edoxaban, rivaroxaban, others) Antiplatelet agents (aspirin, clopidogrel, prasugrel, ticagrelor) Selective serotonin-reuptake inhibitor (SSRI) antidepressants (citalopram, escitalopram, fluoxetine, paroxetine, sertraline)	Bleeding

Red yeast rice	Statin cholesterol medicines (atorvastatin, pravastatin, rosuvastatin, simvastatin, others)	Unexplained muscle pain, kidney damage
St. John's wort	SSRI antidepressants, duloxetine, venlafaxine, trazodone	Increased serotonin levels (symptoms include changes in mental status, increased heart rate, shivering, sweating)
Valerian	Medications that cause drowsiness, such as antianxiety drugs, antidepressants, strong pain medications (opioids), alcohol	Drowsiness, sedation, fall risk

Data that shed light on dietary supplements often come from small studies or even single reports of an adverse event. However, new research and reports continue to be published in the medical literature, which allows our understanding of the safety and effectiveness of various products to evolve. For example, fish oil supplements recently have been associated with an increased risk of atrial fibrillation in some patients.[162] Biotin, a vitamin B supplement, has been reported to interfere with laboratory diagnostic tests for thyroid disorders and heart attacks.[163,164] High doses of turmeric possibly contributed to anemia in a sixty-six-year-old patient.[165] Thus a cautious approach is warranted, and "natural" does not always mean safe.

Mark's story illustrates the potential for a significant interaction with a dietary supplement. He was a seventy-one-year-old gentleman who self-treated with several dietary supplements, one of which was potassium. A relative told him it was good for his heart and blood pressure. However, Mark also was prescribed lisinopril to control his blood pressure. Lisinopril can increase potassium levels. Patient education and warning labels instruct patients to avoid salt substitutes that contain potassium or other potassium supplements unless they are prescribed. Therefore, taking the dietary supplement potassium without talking with his physician was dangerous. Continuing it could have led to high potassium levels, an abnormal heart rhythm, and a possible trip to the emergency department. Potassium supplements, along with calcium and iron, are among the most common supplements associated with emergency department visits.[166]

Another safety issue has to do with the large tablet size of some supplements. Swallowing difficulties were found to contribute to 38 percent of emergency department visits that were caused by dietary supplements among individuals age sixty-five and older. Of note, the FDA is able to regulate tablet size for *drugs*, but no regulations are in place for dietary supplements.[167] Anecdotally, I have seen many patients struggle to swallow large calcium and multivitamin tablets.

One final consideration with dietary supplements is about the quality of manufacturing. As a result of limited federal oversight, there is the risk that a product might contain contaminants, drug ingredients that are not listed on the label, and other impurities that place users at risk.[168,169] This represents another reason for "buyer beware" with supplements. Independent agencies provide testing of dietary supplements to verify product safety and quality. However, this is done only for a fraction of supplements on the market. More information about seals of verification is found in Chapter 18, along with recommendations for choosing a "safer" product.

LABELING AND INSTRUCTIONS FOR USE

Labeling of nonprescription products is regulated by the FDA and is another pertinent consideration for using nonprescription products safely. There are separate label requirements for OTC products and dietary supplements, as shown in **Figures 6-1** and **6-2**. The focus of the labeling requirements is on greater consumer safety. Guidelines have been updated for enhanced readability, simple language, and a standardized format to help consumers find important information. That said, it is important to point out that labeling still might not convey all pertinent information. Seeking the advice of your pharmacist is always recommended as a strategy to prevent unanticipated harm.

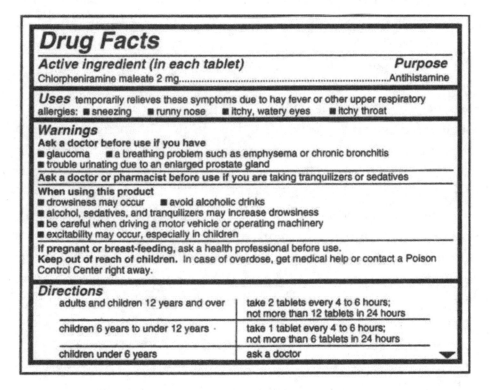

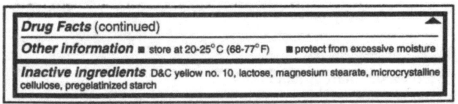

Figure 6-1. Over-the-Counter Drug Facts Label
Source: U.S. Food and Drug Administration

Supplement Facts

Serving Size 1 Capsule

Amount Per Capsule	% Daily Value
Calories 20	
Calories from Fat 20	
Total Fat 2 g	3%*
Saturated Fat 0.5 g	3%*
Polyunsaturated Fat 1 g	†
Monounsaturated Fat 0.5 g	†
Vitamin A 4250 IU	85%
Vitamin D 425 IU	106%
Omega-3 fatty acids 0.5 g	†

* Percent Daily Values are based on a 2,000 calorie diet.
† Daily Value not established.

Ingredients: Cod liver oil, gelatin, water, and glycerin.

Figure 6-2. Supplement Facts Panel
Source: U.S. Food and Drug Administration

The OTC label is officially called the Drug Facts label. In addition to listing the active ingredients and intended use of the product, it must include specific warnings, such as when the drug should be avoided, usually because of interactions; or when to consult with a doctor or pharmacist. It also must include side effects and substances or activities to avoid while taking the product. Unfortunately, these warnings do not always specify important age-related cautions. While the FDA requires labeling to specify issues for pregnant women and children, there is no similar requirement for older adults.[170]

A study published in the *Consultant Pharmacist* in 2018 evaluated the warning information on a sample of fifty OTC products that are associated with important adverse effects in older adults.[171] Researchers found that the labels did not consistently warn older adults about known adverse drug reactions, such as the risk of delirium, confusion, or fall risk. In addition, many warning labels were incomplete or nonspecific with regard to interactions with health conditions, potentially leaving consumers with the impression that the warnings do not apply to them.

Other important information found on the OTC label that consumers should pay attention to is the maximum amount of drug recommended in a twenty-four-hour period and the maximum duration of use. These guidelines are there for safety reasons and should not be disregarded. Taking more than is recommended is not safe, and if symptoms persist or worsen once the recommended duration is reached (when provided), it is important to seek medical attention and not continue to self-treat.

The official name for the dietary supplement label is the Supplement Facts panel, which must include the names and quantities of the ingredients. Remember that dietary supplements are regulated as foods by the FDA; thus, similar to food labels, the Supplement Facts panel must include information about calories, fat, and vitamin content. The first line of the Supplement Facts panel states the "serving size," an important but often overlooked piece of information. The serving size is the rough equivalent to the "active ingredient" portion of the Drug Facts label, where the ingredient amount per each tablet or capsule is listed. Products like calcium citrate or fish oil preparations often have a serving size of two tablets, for example. Buyers need to beware that the dietary supplement packaging can be misleading because the stated amount on the front of the package often implies the amount per *serving size*, which might be different than the amount *per tablet* (for example, 1000 mg is stated on the front, but the serving size is two tablets with 500 mg per tablet).

MULTIPLE INGREDIENT PRODUCTS

There are many OTC products and dietary supplements on the market that contain multiple ingredients. Using multi-ingredient products increases the risk of being exposed to additional and often unnecessary drug interactions and side effects. Products that include ingredients of questionable value should be avoided. During the course of a consultation with me, older adults and their family members often are surprised to learn that their nonprescription products contain "hidden" drugs they had no idea they were taking.

Of particular concern with multi-ingredient products is the risk of overdosing on an ingredient that is contained in multiple products. An important example of this is with acetaminophen (Tylenol®). Acetaminophen can cause liver damage when use exceeds the maximum amount recommended in a twenty-four-hour period. Acetaminophen is an ingredient in over six hundred prescription and OTC products in the United States, including products to self-treat pain, sleep issues, and cough and cold symptoms.[172] Acetaminophen also is contained in combination-ingredient prescription pain medications. As a result, patients who ingest acetaminophen from different sources can end up taking more than the safe amount without realizing it. Acetaminophen used alone or in combination products accounts for 44 percent of medication errors involving pain medicines.[173]

On the dietary supplement side, products frequently contain multiple herbal ingredients or proprietary blends that do not specify the separate ingredients. In these cases, it can be challenging if not impossible to evaluate potential drug interactions. For many herbal products there simply are no data available to clinicians to inform decisions about safe use of the supplement.

BRAND-NAME EXTENSIONS AND CONFUSING PACKAGING FOR OTC PRODUCTS

A unique caveat for OTC products is the presence of brand-name extension products. This marketing technique can deceive consumers into choosing a product they are familiar with, but that actually contains a different ingredient. Examples of brand-name extension products are found in **Table 6-6**.[174] Note the difference in ingredients between the original products and the extension products with the modified name. With brand-name extension products, manufacturers use a trusted brand name that is associated with one ingredient, but then extend the brand name to market additional products that contain either an added ingredient or altogether different active ingredients. This can lead to medication errors and adverse outcomes when individuals choose the wrong product. Look-alike packaging and distracting words further add to the confusion. Choosing Tylenol PM® instead of Tylenol®, for example, can be deleterious to an older adult. To combat the potential for confusion, consumers need to use the OTC Drug Facts label and, when in doubt, double check with a pharmacist to confirm they have chosen the product with the proper ingredients.

Table 6-6. Examples of Brand-Name Extension of OTC Products

Original (familiar) brand name	Active ingredient in original product	Extension product name	Active ingredient(s) in extension product
Aleve®	Naproxen	Aleve® Arthritis Pain Gel	Diclofenac
Zantac®	Ranitidine*	Zantac 360°®	Famotidine
Dulcolax®	Bisacodyl	Dulcolax® Stool Softener	Docusate sodium
Mucinex®	Guaifenesin	Mucinex Sinus-Max® Night	Acetaminophen, dextromethorphan, doxylamine, and phenylephrine
Sudafed®	Pseudoephedrine	Sudafed PE®	Phenylephrine
Tylenol®	Acetaminophen	Tylenol PM®	Acetaminophen and diphenhydramine

*Ranitidine was withdrawn from the market in 2020.

SUMMARY

OTC drugs and dietary supplements are widely used as self-care options by older adults. The majority of patients mix nonprescription products with prescription drugs but do not consistently share this information with their physicians. OTC products and dietary supplements need to be included on every individual's medication list alongside the prescribed medications.

Nonprescription products should be regarded with the same level of respect as prescribed drugs. Unnecessary use and misuse should be avoided to reduce the risk of an adverse drug event. While OTC drugs and dietary supplements are an important part of the self-care movement and can be effective tools for managing one's health, these products carry risks when not used properly. Pharmacists are excellent resources to guide consumers on the selection and use of OTC drugs and dietary supplements. Strategies and tips to improve the safe use nonprescription products are provided in Chapter 18.

KEY POINTS

- OTC drugs and dietary supplements are available without a prescription; however, they are not necessarily safer than prescription drugs, especially if they are taken in a manner different than the labeled instructions and warnings.
- Both OTC drugs and dietary supplements need to be included as part of a complete medication list; they can have side effects and drug interactions similar to prescription medications.
- OTC products have the potential to cause important interactions for older adults; however, product labeling might be vague or incomplete.
- Dietary supplements are regulated as foods by the FDA, rather than as drugs. This has important implications for the safety and effectiveness of these products.

Chapter 7

Nondrug Treatment Strategies to Manage Health Conditions

Previous chapters have described concerns associated with use of excessive and unnecessary medications. Thus, it is important to appreciate that there is much we can do to improve our health and well-being by looking beyond prescriptions as our only solution. Medications have a valuable and necessary role in keeping us healthy and extending lives. However, for many health conditions, medications are only part of the solution. Nondrug treatments refer to health-care interventions that do not involve medications or pharmaceuticals. Another term is nonpharmacologic treatments, but I will stick with the simpler word "nondrug."

Nondrug treatment strategies can help manage symptoms and offer long-term health benefits. This topic matters and needs to be included in this book because ultimately, incorporating nondrug treatment strategies offers the opportunity to reduce polypharmacy (use of multiple medications) and adverse drug events. These strategies should be included in conversation with your health-care team about treatment options. Unfortunately, these "other" options often are minimized or overlooked. Thus, it falls to the patient or family member to start the conversation and ask about nondrug options when faced with a new diagnosis or symptom.

What do individuals need to know about nondrug treatment strategies, and how can they integrate this information into the larger goal of using medications more safely? This chapter will provide an overview and general guidance. Nondrug treatment strategies is a broad topic, and this chapter can only scratch the surface of it. Readers are encouraged to continue to explore and learn about nondrug options from trusted experts.

WHAT ARE NONDRUG TREATMENT STRATEGIES?

Nondrug treatments include a broad array of interventions. Common examples are described later in the chapter and are listed in **Table 7-1**. Lifestyle modifications include healthy behaviors, such as eating a healthy diet, getting regular physical activity, and quitting smoking. They also include health condition-specific recommendations; for example, to manage reflux symptoms, individuals can adjust the timing and size of meals and elevate the head of their bed, along with other recommendations. These types of disease-specific modifications sometimes are referred to as "therapeutic lifestyle changes." Other nondrug options simply offer alternatives to drug therapy; for example, applying heat or cold to manage pain or getting physical therapy.

Table 7-1. Examples of Nondrug Treatments

Nondrug approaches	Examples

Lifestyle Modifications	• Healthy behaviors
	  ○ Healthy diet, nutrition
	  ○ Exercise, physical activity
	  ○ Smoking cessation
	  ○ Limit alcohol intake
	  ○ Weight management/weight loss
	  ○ Social engagement
	  ○ Sleep health
	• Therapeutic lifestyle changes (health condition-specific recommendations)
	  ○ Sleep hygiene for insomnia, recommendations for managing reflux symptoms or managing constipation

Complementary or Alternative Medicine (mind and body approaches)	• Acupuncture • Cognitive behavioral therapy • Chiropractic • Massage • Meditation • Relaxation • Tai Chi • Yoga
Conventional Medicine	• Physical therapy

Long-term healthy behaviors make up the core of disease prevention and healthy aging and can be adopted at any age, although earlier always is better. Robust data show that healthy lifestyle behaviors can slow, prevent, and, in some cases, even reverse disease progression. Benefits of these lifestyle modifications are described in more detail later in the chapter.

Complementary and alternative medicine (CAM) refers to interventions that are not part of conventional medical practice. CAM includes mind-body therapies like meditation, relaxation, and Tai Chi. Dietary supplements often are considered as CAM. However, for the purposes of this book, I have chosen to group them with nonprescription medications in the previous chapter.

Physical therapy is somewhat of an outlier among nondrug strategies in that it is accessed within conventional medical practice and typically is covered by insurance. Along with other nondrug approaches, it can reduce or avoid the need for long-term drug therapy.

ROLE OF NONDRUG TREATMENTS

Nondrug treatments have a role in managing many health conditions. They can be used alone or in addition to drug therapy and other medical approaches, depending on the particular health condition. Indeed, it is not unreasonable to start a nondrug treatment strategy before moving to drug therapy, in hopes of improving the signs or symptoms of the health condition without need for a medication. For example, diet modification, physical activity, and achieving a healthy weight are essential first steps in the management of diabetes, high blood pressure, high cholesterol, and other cardiovascular conditions.

There is specific terminology for CAM therapies, depending on how they are applied to one's health care. CAM treatments that are used *instead of* conventional medicine are defined as alternative therapies. When they are used *in conjunction with* conventional medicine, they are defined as complementary or integrative therapies. Many CAM therapies are used in either capacity, and thus referring to them as "CAM" is most simple. For example, when treating mild depression in older adults, cognitive behavioral therapy (CBT) is recommended as initial therapy, but it can be combined with antidepressant drug therapy, as well.[175] Treatments that center on lifestyle modifications like diet and exercise frequently are integrated as part of the standard of care for a number of diagnoses. Importantly, positive lifestyle changes should always be continued, even once drug therapy is initiated. Making these changes part of your way of life can yield long-term benefits by slowing disease progression and the need for additional drug therapy.

Many chronic health conditions are caused by unhealthy lifestyle choices, which make healthy behaviors an especially important topic for everyone interested in healthy aging. Data from the Centers for Disease Control and Prevention (CDC) show that cardiovascular disease is the number one cause of death in older adults.[176] Roughly 45 percent of adults age sixty-five to seventy-four years are obese;[177] and more than one in four older adults (27 percent) have diabetes.[178] Adopting healthy behaviors, primarily a healthy diet and being physically active, can reduce these statistics and improve health outcomes. Perhaps the most notable testament to this is the significant improvement in the control of type 2 diabetes that can be achieved through diet, exercise, and weight management interventions, often reducing the need for drug therapy.[179]

Not to be outdone by lifestyle choices, CAM options also can be extremely beneficial and help patients reduce or avoid the need for drug therapy. Mind and body approaches can improve stress, mental health, balance, and strength, for example. The struggle is to get effective CAM options to be more widely acknowledged, recommended by clinicians, and paid for by insurance companies. Barriers that contribute to the poor uptake of proven CAM therapies are described later. **Table 7-2** lists some examples of nondrug treatment strategies that are supported by scientific evidence and have a role in managing various health conditions commonly seen in older adults.[180,181,182]

Table 7-2. Nondrug Treatment Strategies Specific to Selected Health Conditions

Health condition	Selected recommended nondrug treatments (lists are not complete)
Coronary artery disease	• Healthy diet • Regular physical activity (aerobic exercise) • Smoking cessation • Weight reduction in obese individuals
Chronic obstructive pulmonary disease (COPD)	• Smoking cessation
Constipation	• Increase fluid intake and dietary fiber • Engage in physical activity to help bowel regularity
Diabetes	• Dietary modification (medical nutrition therapy) • Regular physical activity (such as walking) • Achieve healthy weight

Gastrointestinal reflux disease (GERD)	• Avoid food irritants (such as spicy foods, coffee, citrus juices) • Smoking cessation • Achieve healthy weight
Pain, chronic (including osteoarthritis)	• Set reasonable goals focused on improved functioning • Exercise, Tai Chi, heat or cold therapy, acupuncture • Physical therapy, occupational therapy
Sleep disorder	• Practice good sleep hygiene (limit naps; avoid large, late meals; avoid caffeine after noon, avoid alcohol before bedtime) • Cognitive behavioral therapy for insomnia (CBT-I)

Carl offers an example of the success associated with healthy behavior changes. Carl was seventy-seven years old when I met with him. He had high blood pressure, high cholesterol, and diabetes. One of his concerns was occasional episodes of low blood sugar (hypoglycemia). He was taking valsartan for blood pressure, atorvastatin for cholesterol, and metformin and glipizide for diabetes. Carl shared with me his accomplishments over the past two years of starting a routine of exercising five days a week; shifting away from a diet of junk food, fast food, and processed meat; and losing fifty pounds. He was proud of his accomplishments, and deservedly so. As a result of these meaningful and sustained changes, Carl's blood sugar control improved significantly. His diabetes medications essentially were too strong for him now and contributed to low blood sugar levels. His physician was able to reduce Carl's diabetes medications and stop one of them altogether.

BENEFITS OF NONDRUG TREATMENTS

No medication is totally risk-free. Therefore, one of the key benefits of nondrug treatments is that in many cases they offer a way to delay or reduce the reliance on drug therapy. In turn, this can reduce the number of medicines an individual needs to take and reduce the chance of an adverse reaction, interaction, or another medication-related problem. As mentioned earlier, adopting healthy behaviors (healthy diet, exercise, quitting smoking, etc.) makes it possible to reduce the need for medications when significant and sustained efforts are made, as Carl's story illustrates.

Nondrug treatment strategies play an important role in improving mind and body health and an overall sense of well-being. Tai Chi, for example, can improve pain and daily functioning.[183] Exercise and physical therapy for patients with Parkinson's disease can improve stability and reduce fall risk.[184] Nondrug strategies can improve quality of life when an individual has fewer pills to take each day and a lower risk of side effects. In addition, medication costs can be reduced, both for an individual and from an insurance payer's perspective.

The benefits and importance of adopting healthy behaviors warrants particular attention by everyone who wants to age in a healthful manner. Healthy diet, physical activity, not smoking, limiting alcohol, and maintaining a healthy weight are the mainstay behaviors for optimizing health and promoting healthy aging (listed in **Table 7-1**). These are key strategies that should be broadly embedded in health care priorities, especially in light of our aging population.[185] Two additional behaviors are gathering momentum regarding their role in healthy aging: sleep health[186,187] and social isolation.[188]

Physical activity or exercise is promoted as one of the most effective modifiable risk factors to promote healthy aging. Exercise as medicine is a growing reality. It reduces the risk of heart disease, diabetes, dementia, falls, and other maladies.[189] There is a growing appreciation of the role of exercise to manage pain,[190] and it is a mainstay therapy to improve diabetes, blood pressure, and weight management.[191,192] Studies indicate that exercise or some level of physical activity is possible for just about every older adult, regardless of physical and cognitive function. Thus, older adults are encouraged to talk with their physicians about physical activity options that are safe and appropriate for them.

Independently, each healthy behavior is beneficial, but they have even greater benefit when combined. The core triad of a healthy diet, regular physical activity, and not smoking has been frequently studied in combination with one or more additional healthy behaviors. A range of positive outcomes has been documented. Research specifically in older adults shows benefits of increased longevity and reduced mortality, as well as reduced risk of heart disease, stroke, diabetes, and dementia.[193,194,195,196] Studies also show that more lifestyle modifications are better than fewer. Patients who adopt four or five healthy behaviors experience even greater benefit than patients who adopt only three.[197] Importantly, taking multiple medications (polypharmacy) does not take away from this benefit. In one study, individuals with an average age of sixty-five benefited from a reduced mortality risk regardless of the number of medications they took.[198] Thus, even older adults with multiple health conditions who take ten or more medications are encouraged to continue their healthy lifestyle choices.[199]

More good news is that adopting healthy behaviors shows benefit even when adopted later in life. Apparently, it is never too late to make a change. Several studies have looked at modifications in patients into their eighties. A sampling of the findings is listed here:

- Men who maintained healthy behaviors at age seventy-one were found to maintain their cognitive and physical function at age eighty-five.[200]
- Beginning a physical activity program at an average age of seventy-nine was found to help a group of individuals maintain their mobility and level of physical functioning almost three years later.[201]
- Patients over the age of sixty with diabetes who made lifestyle changes had a lower risk of developing cardiovascular disease and death.[202]
- Smokers who quit after age sixty experienced reduced risk of stroke, heart disease, and heart-related deaths within five years of quitting.[203]

Healthy behaviors as a subset of nondrug treatment strategies are a powerful and important topic when discussing healthy aging. We need to look no further than the current status of heart disease, diabetes, and obesity in our society to know we can do better. **Table 7-3** lists several resources for older adults that address healthy behaviors. As mentioned earlier, this chapter can only scratch the surface, and readers are encouraged to discuss healthy behaviors as well as other nondrug treatment strategies with their health-care professionals.

BARRIERS TO NONDRUG TREATMENTS

Despite expert consensus that nondrug treatments have a valid role in managing health conditions and in disease prevention, why are these options not more widely discussed and promoted during health-care encounters? The following describes several barriers at play that hinder greater acceptance of these "other" treatment options.

To begin with, the health culture in the United States is focused on medications, which are associated with quick and easy fixes. We live in a pill-for-every-ill culture, and nondrug options require considerable time and effort. It is harder to prepare a healthy meal compared to picking up something from the nearest fast-food restaurant. It takes a lot of discipline and support to quit smoking. Physical therapy exercises need to be practiced in between sessions.

Patients also want immediate results. The onset of effect of medications is relatively quick compared to months or years for some lifestyle changes. Furthermore, the goals of lifestyle changes often are to prevent a health condition, such as diabetes; or prevent an event, such as a stroke or heart attack. These goals require a long-term commitment and persistent motivation. On top of this, success in achieving these goals is measured by the absence of the condition or event—something that cannot be pinpointed but certainly is worth celebrating.

Nondrug treatments are more expensive and harder to access. Many older adults are saddled with financial and geographic limitations. Fresh fruits, vegetables, and fish are more expensive than processed foods and are not consistently available. Individuals who have mobility issues or do not drive may not be able to get to the grocery store or an exercise class on a regular basis. There is a growing awareness of inequities in health care that are directly impacted by where one lives. For many individuals, accessing good nutrition, a safe place to exercise, and even access to medical care, let alone some of the CAM options, can be challenging if not impossible.

Insurance coverage certainly impacts acceptance of nondrug treatments. For example, traditional Medicare will cover smoking cessation programs, physical therapy, and nutrition education in certain situations,[204] but therapies like Tai Chi, massage, or gym memberships likely are out-of-pocket expenses. Coverage through Medicare Advantage plans might differ, but further discussion is beyond the scope of this chapter. In addition, some of the specialized therapies, such as cognitive behavioral therapy for insomnia (CBT-I), requires clinicians who are specifically trained in this technique. In certain geographic regions, there might not be anyone who has the official training.

Another barrier is the lack of research on the effectiveness of CAM treatments. Clinicians do not always know how a CAM option stacks up to traditional drug therapy or if it is effective in older individuals. Many studies are small or of short duration, which makes it difficult to know when an option might be a good choice for an individual.

Physicians can be barriers to nondrug treatments if they lack sufficient knowledge to address these options with their patients. Most medical training programs provide only minimal education on nutrition, for example.[205] As a result, physicians might be less comfortable starting a conversation with patients about dietary changes. In addition, physicians and other prescribers who lack sufficient geriatric training might not appreciate the potential for increased risk of harm associated with certain medications. As a result, they are more ready to prescribe medications rather than consider viable nondrug options.

Furthermore, physicians are trained to make people feel better, and patients often expect direct fixes to their problems. Prescribing a new medication fits the bill for a quick and easy solution compared to developing a step-by-step plan with the patient for how to lose weight, for example.

This point is illustrated clearly in a story relayed by an ophthalmologist colleague. He saw one of his patients for a routine diabetic eye exam. At one point during the encounter, the patient commented about his diabetes drug, "Yeah, my doctor said that if this medication doesn't lower my blood sugar enough, I'll have to go on a diet." The eye doctor was stunned. "But that's totally backwards!" he replied.

Finally, the current reimbursement model for physicians is a barrier to promoting nondrug treatments. Discussing and exploring nondrug options with a patient takes time. Physicians in busy practices often have only limited time to spend with each patient, and unfortunately, they may not be able to bill the health insurance company for time spent on these conversations.

PATIENT ROLE IN INCORPORATING NONDRUG TREATMENTS

Nondrug treatments are an essential part of the care plan for most health conditions, but they often take a back seat to conventional drug therapy. Physicians might not bring up these options when discussing treatment choices for the previously mentioned reasons. So, what is your role in incorporating nondrug treatments into your overall health-care plan?

First, bring up the topic when discussing ways to manage your health conditions, especially for a new condition. What lifestyle changes can you make that might be helpful and reduce the need for drug therapy? Is there evidence that a CAM treatment might be effective?

To illustrate the value of exploring nondrug options, Miriam's story is important. She was eighty-eight years old and quite healthy except for high blood pressure and occasional lower back pain. One day she awoke with worsened back pain, severe enough she went to her doctor, who pre-scribed carisoprodol (Soma®), a muscle relaxer. Taking this medication for three days led to such extreme sedation that Miriam had trouble with her speech and was unable to carry out her usual daily routine at home. At one point, she fell when trying to get out of bed. Worst of all, the medication did not take away the pain; it merely made her tired enough to sleep. She ultimately recovered, but not before in-home care was needed for a few days.

Her internist sadly had missed the chance to discuss safer and likely more effective nondrug options with Miriam. Miriam, like most individuals, did not know to ask about these options, unaware of the potential harm of the muscle relaxer. If she had brought up the question of nondrug alternatives with her doctor, she possibly could have avoided the sequence of adverse events.

Another role you have regarding nondrug strategies is to make sure your health-care team knows if you are using any of these options, especially CAM. Two-thirds of patients do not tell their physicians.[206] There is no harm in sharing this information, and it can help your physician understand what you value in health care and provide more person-centered care. If you prefer a nondrug treatment over conventional drug therapy, talk to your physician to find out what is known about the effectiveness and potential harms of the treatment you have in mind. Not all CAM approaches have been studied or are effective. The downside is that choosing a CAM approach that is of questionable benefit can be harmful to your health; especially if you forego a conventional treatment that is of known benefit.

The lifelong benefits of incorporating nondrug treatments into your daily routine are immense and include physical, cognitive, and emotional well-being. This mostly applies to the various lifestyle modifications, but many of the mind-body CAM examples listed in **Table 7-1** theoretically have long-term benefits, too. Recognize that change is difficult and old lifestyle habits are hard to break, so be patient. Don't give up. Make sure you have a support network of family and friends, in addition to your health-care team.

Be informed about lifestyle modifications (healthy behaviors) and what the guidelines are for older adults. Resources for additional information are provided in **Table 7-3**. While all of these behaviors are important, I want to emphasize the importance of being aware of changes in nutritional recommendations for older adults. For example, there is a greater emphasis on sufficient hydration (fluids) and protein intake and on foods that are nutrient-rich (as opposed to sweets that are high in calories but low in nutrients). My Plate for Older Adults provides age-specific guidelines (see **Table 7-3**).

Table 7-3. Resources on Healthy Behaviors for Older Adults

Category	Online Resource
Diet	• USDA My Plate for Older Adults: https://www .myplate.gov/life-stages/older-adults • MyPlate Plan: https://www.myplate.gov/myplate-plan (personalized food plan based on age, sex, height, weight, and physical activity level) • Nutrition as We Age: Healthy Eating with the Dietary Guidelines, https://health.gov/news/202107 /nutrition-we-age-healthy-eating-dietary-guidelines • Healthy Meal Planning: Tips for Older Adults, https://www.nia.nih.gov/health /healthy-meal-planning-tips-older-adults
Exercise/physical activity	• Making physical activity a part of an older adult's life: https://www.cdc.gov/physicalactivity/basics/adding-pa/ activities-olderadults.htm • Exercise and physical activity: https://www.nia.nih .gov/health/exercise-physical-activity • Exercise for Older Adults: https://medlineplus.gov /exerciseforolderadults.html • The Life-changing Benefits of Exercise After 60: https://www.ncoa.org/article /the-life-changing-benefits-of-exercise-after-60
Smoking cessation	• National Institute on Aging: Quit Smoking for Older Adults, https://www.nia.nih.gov/health (under Smoking in A-Z Health Topics) • Smoke Free 60+: https://60plus.smokefree.gov/

Alcohol use	• Alcohol Use or Abuse: https://www.nia.nih.gov/health/topics/alcohol-use-or-abuse • Older Adults, National Institute on Alcohol Abuse and Alcoholism: https://www.niaaa.nih.gov/alcohols-effects-health/special-populations-co-occurring-disorders/older-adults
Sleep Health	• National Institute on Aging: A Good Night's Sleep, https://www.nia.nih.gov/health/good-nights-sleep • Medline Plus: Aging Changes in Sleep, https://medlineplus.gov/ency/article/004018.htm
Social Isolation	• Centers for Disease Control and Prevention (CDC): Loneliness and Social Isolation Linked to Serious Health Conditions, https://www.cdc.gov/aging/publications/features/lonely-older-adults.html • National Health Service (UK): Loneliness in Older People, https://www.nhs.uk/mental-health/feelings-symptoms-behaviours/feelings-and-symptoms/loneliness-in-older-people/

Of course, there are cautions to consider. Talk with your physicians before starting a nondrug treatment. Make sure it is safe and effective for your situation and works well with your conventional medicine treatment plan. Check first with your doctor before beginning an exercise program. It is important to choose the right type of activity and intensity to make sure it is a safe undertaking. Similarly, talk with your doctor and ideally a nutritionist before attempting to lose weight. As we get older, weight loss must be approached more carefully to ensure sufficient protein and nutrient intake to avoid loss of muscle mass.[207] This chapter cannot cover all concerns, and everyone's situation is different. Therefore, it is important to consult with your physician about these and other nondrug treatment strategies.

SUMMARY

The information in this chapter provides a general overview of the types of nondrug options that are available. Ideally, nondrug treatment strategies allow for reduced reliance on medications and healthier aging. These options tend to be more challenging to implement due to various barriers. They require greater time and effort by both the provider and patient, health insurance typically does not pay for these services, and most are not well-studied. Seven healthy behaviors are a particularly important subset of nondrug treatments and are an essential aspect of healthy and independent aging.

Nondrug treatment options should be included in every discussion of how to best manage a health condition. If physicians do not bring up the topic, older adults and their family members are encouraged to do so. Medications have an important role in our health and well-being, but we need to do a better job of incorporating nondrug treatment strategies to improve health outcomes and ideally reduce our reliance on medications where possible.

KEY POINTS

- Nondrug treatments include lifestyle modifications such as diet, exercise, and smoking cessation; and complementary and alternative treatments such as acupuncture, cognitive behavioral therapy, and massage.
- Nondrug options should be included in the discussion of how to manage new symptoms or a new diagnosis.
- Barriers that prevent the widespread adoption of nondrug treatments include time, effort, cost, accessibility, and limited knowledge and awareness.
- Benefits of lifestyle modifications can be realized even later in life. It is never too late to make healthier choices.

Part IV

Medication Issues that Matter Most to Older Adults

Chapter 8

Medication Adherence

Medications are one of the most important treatment options we have for managing chronic health conditions. However, if patients do not take their medications, or do not take them in the correct manner, they will not work. The term "medication adherence" is defined in more detail soon, but in short, it refers to taking medications as instructed. Nonadherence is the flip side; that is, not taking one's medications as instructed. While it sounds so simple on the surface, adherence is a huge concern for individuals of all ages, particularly among older adults. This concept is at the core of effective drug therapy and should be a matter of high importance to anyone who is prescribed medications. Yet, surprisingly, problems with adherence are not readily obvious to clinicians and patients alike: unless we ask about adherence, it typically doesn't come up.

Medication adherence is a behavior, just like exercising daily or eating vegetables. As with most behaviors, we make a choice to adopt that behavior or not. Many factors can impact the ability of a person to adhere to a drug regimen (the medication treatment plan). Importantly, it is not just the patient's problem to deal with. Good medication adherence requires the input of different members of the health-care team, including the patient. Family members often are involved and play a supportive role in helping to manage complex medicine schedules and follow correct instructions.

The problem of nonadherence falls within the medication-related problem (MRP) category of not receiving a medication, described in Chapter 3. Thus, medication adherence (or more aptly, nonadherence) is a preventable problem. This chapter provides information on why this topic matters to older adults along with general guidance on how to improve adherence. In turn, patients and consumers are empowered to achieve better management of their health conditions. Chapter 17 is closely related and focuses on ways to address specific barriers to adherence.

DEFINITION

Medication adherence is defined as the extent to which individuals take medications according to the agreed-upon recommendations from their health-care providers. You might be familiar with "compliance," which is the older term. Compliance is no longer favored because it implies a passive role in which patients are expected simply to follow a doctor's medication instructions without question. In contrast, adherence is the newer term and preferred because it embodies a collaborative spirit between patient and physician. It acknowledges that patients have choices regarding their medications, and the responsibility for taking them as instructed never falls solely on the patient. Adherence implies that patients and physicians are in agreement with treatment recommendations based on what is most important for the patient. "Persistence" is yet another term that refers to ongoing adherence over time. Medication persistence matters with long-term (chronic) medical conditions such as asthma, diabetes, or high blood pressure for which drug therapy needs to be continued, usually for years. Low persistence is a particular concern when treating health conditions that lack symptoms, such as high cholesterol or osteoporosis.

There are many ways in which patients might not adhere to their medication regimens. Nonadherence can be intentional or unintentional (see **Box 8-1**). Unintentional nonadherence occurs when individuals are unaware of their mistakes in following the medication instructions. I met with one client who simply forgot to get his new diabetes medicine refilled and thus quit taking it unintentionally. Another client took her once-weekly alendronate to treat osteoporosis every Sunday with lunch. She was confident that she was taking it correctly, but did not understand that she needed to take it on an empty stomach, thirty minutes before breakfast or other medications.

Box 8-1. Examples of Ways in which Patients Are Not Adherent with Their Medications

- Failing to get a medication refilled
- Skipping a dose on purpose to save money or because of side effects
- Stopping a medication because you "feel fine"
- Stopping a medication because you don't think it is needed
- Taking someone else's medication
- Forgetting to take a medication dose
- Taking more medication or less medication than prescribed
- Not using an inhaler or eye drops correctly
- Taking medications with food or beverage that should be avoided
- Taking medication at the wrong time of day

Another common cause of unintentional nonadherence is not taking the time to read the instructions on the prescription label carefully. I have had clients tell me they take a drug once daily when the label states to take it twice daily. They then admit to not having read the label carefully. Unclear instructions can lead to unintentional nonadherence, as well. Errors can occur when patients interpret "two times daily" as taking both tablets together as one dose in the morning, rather taking one tablet at two different times of the day (such as morning and evening). Several of my clients have misinterpreted what the phrase "as needed" means. For example, they understood "Take three times a day as needed" to mean they should take the medicine three times a day, regardless of whether the symptom the drug is treating is present or not. "It must be needed if the doctor prescribed it," they explained.

Intentional nonadherence occurs when people knowingly do not take their medications as instructed and reportedly occurs more frequently than unintentional nonadherence.[208] There are many ways in which people might knowingly not take their medications as instructed. Some might intentionally stop a medication because they believe it is not needed, they heard something negative through social media, or they read something on the internet that concerned them. Other individuals skip doses on purpose to save money or because of side effects. As an aside, having side effects actually could be a valid reason to be intentionally nonadherent—however, not without talking to your health-care professional about it. Stopping medicines abruptly can be dangerous. Of note, some side effects are mild and easily manageable or they might go away with time.

A person can be fully adherent, partially adherent, or nonadherent. It is not uncommon for individuals to have mixed levels of adherence, meaning they might be fully adherent with some medications and nonadherent with others. This can be referred to as partial adherence, which is reported to occur in about 30 percent of adults.[209] Charles is one of my clients who illustrates partial adherence. He was prescribed four oral medications to manage diabetes, high blood pressure, and urinary symptoms of an enlarged prostate. He also had prescriptions for two inhalers to manage chronic obstructive pulmonary disease (COPD). Charles was great about taking his oral medications every day. However, he had not refilled one of the inhalers in over four months because he did not think it was necessary.

Nonadherence is never encouraged, of course, and can lead to serious health problems. Occasionally I have met with clients who either never started or they stopped taking a medication after just a few days. Rather than making a decision like this on your own, speak with your physician or pharmacist first. Stopping a medication on your own or taking it in a manner other than how it is prescribed is risky. Abruptly discontinuing a drug, even if just for a few days, can lead to other adverse events. For example, stopping blood pressure medications can lead to rebound increased blood pressure and the risk of a stroke; certain antidepressants can cause withdrawal symptoms if stopped suddenly. As a general rule of safety, individuals should never stop a medication without first checking with their physician or pharmacist.

IMPORTANCE OF MEDICATION ADHERENCE

Fran asked to meet with me because she had concerns about her medications. "I'm sure I am having side effects because I'm not taking my medicines correctly," she said. "Pills fall on the floor, so I reach for another one to replace it and I'm not sure I'm taking the correct medicine." Her medication bottles were spread across the kitchen table. Among them were open bottles and three pill organizers of varying sizes. One of them had an unexplained mix of tablets and capsules in random compartments. She readily admitted that she didn't know how to organize her medicines and when to take them. Fran was struggling with adherence. Her health conditions were not well-controlled, and some of her "side effects" likely were related to worsening health. She was spending money on unnecessary refills and prescriptions she no longer needed.

Fran did not know the reasons for several of her medications. She believed many were not needed and causing side effects. Fran's knowledge of and beliefs about her medications were having a direct impact on her adherence. To help Fran better understand how her medications may or may not be affecting her health and causing some of her symptoms, I sorted through each one with her. I explained which were essential for managing her chronic health conditions and thus needed to be continued and which were prescribed to treat specific symptoms or short-term conditions (like for treating allergies or pain, for example). These types of drugs often are less critical; based on her preferences, she could talk with her doctor about reducing them. I identified other medications for which it was unclear why she was taking them and whether they still were needed. In the end, Fran had a better knowledge of her medications and why each was prescribed; she could focus on regularly taking the essential ones on a regular basis and use her pill organizer correctly to help her remember to take them. Importantly, she scheduled an appointment to speak with her physician about possibly stopping some of the other drug therapy.

Drug therapy has tremendous value in managing chronic health conditions. It prevents diseases from getting worse, improves symptoms and quality of life, and ultimately extends lives. However, medications cannot help patients who do not take them correctly or who stop taking them, as Fran experienced. Therefore, medication adherence is a critical component of staying healthy as we age.

Adherence rates are dismal, however. It is estimated that roughly 50 percent of older adults have some level of nonadherence to their drug regimens.[210,211,212] Across all age groups, nearly one in four individuals never even fill a new prescription.[213] In one study of community-dwelling older adults, the rate of full adherence to several types of long-term medications was barely 20 percent.[214] Over one-third had poor adherence to at least one of their long-term medications.[215]

Costs of nonadherence are significant at both the personal and societal levels. Adherence is of particular concern in older adults because there is a greater reliance on medications to manage more chronic conditions compared to a younger population. As a result, individuals who do not take their medications properly are at higher risk of their health conditions worsening. Poor control of the signs or symptoms the medications were prescribed to treat can lead to the need for added medications, more laboratory testing to monitor drug therapy, extra outpatient clinic visits, and emergency department visits or even hospitalization.[216,217] Costs at the societal level are significant in terms of dollars and the need for higher levels of care:

- $100 to $300 billion in health-care expenditures[218]
- 125,000 preventable deaths[219]
- 10 to 26 percent of hospitalizations among older adults[220,221]
- 23 percent of nursing home admissions[222]

Thus, we need to be vigilant about poor adherence and continue efforts to identify and remove barriers to help older individuals age healthily and independently.

There are no good clues that help us predict which individuals will be adherent to their medications. Age alone generally is not a factor, nor is one's education level.[223] An older adult is equally able to take a medication correctly compared to a younger person. Problems arise when several medications need to be taken multiple times a day and with specific instructions.[224] Once-daily medications are associated with three-fold better adherence rates compared to medicines that must be taken two or more times per day.[225]

Physical and cognitive changes can complicate adherence efforts. For example, vision changes can affect the ability to read instructions on the label or differentiate tablet size and color. Changes in dexterity and hand strength can make it difficult to open medication bottles and manipulate small tablets. Decreased hearing can impact the ability to correctly understand information provided verbally. Other challenges are present for individuals who experience decreased memory and dementia.[226] A study published in 2014 in the *Annals of Pharmacotherapy* showed that complex drug regimens are associated with an increased risk of hospitalization.[227] Thus, working with a pharmacist to simplify one's drug regimen has the potential to improve adherence and health outcomes. Better yet, requesting a medication review to identify medications that might be reduced or stopped can also improve adherence by decreasing the number of medications and undue financial burden.

Unfortunately, poor medication adherence is rarely obvious and not a focus during patient-physician encounters. Nonadherence is difficult to detect, and patients generally do not volunteer to their physician or pharmacist that they have not been taking a medication. There are understandable reasons for this. When adherence is unintentional, people are not aware there is a problem. On the other hand, patients who know they are nonadherent may not want to upset or disappoint their physician because they are not following instructions. Some might be embarrassed about their nonadherence; for example, when cost is a problem. Others may not want to admit they are forgetful in case it is sign of a more serious problem. Thus, to our detriment, nonadherence typically hovers under the radar until a problem occurs or the patient's condition deteriorates. It often is only at that point that a thorough medication review uncovers adherence issues that can be addressed.

BARRIERS TO MEDICATION ADHERENCE

There are myriad factors that can get in the way of medication adherence. We refer to these as adherence barriers. Barriers can be grouped into five general categories: patient-related, health condition–related, medication-related, finance-related, and health-care–system related. Examples of each category are provided in **Table 8-1**.[228,229,230] Many of these barriers are beyond a patient's control, such as medication costs or poor communication with the health-care provider. Subsequently, a patient who is nonadherent should never be blamed. The most common reasons older adults cite for not adhering to their medications are as follows:[231,232]

- Belief the drug is not effective
- Belief the drug is not needed
- Adverse effects or side effects
- Forgetting to take the drug
- Physical barriers, such as low vision or arthritis
- Cost of the medication
- Confusion about when or how to take the medication
- Illnesses that have no symptoms and thus no cues that a medication is needed

Many of these reasons can be addressed through better communication and collaboration.

Table 8-1. Adherence Barriers

Category of barrier	Common examples
Related to patient	Forgetfulness Not understanding the medication or disease Belief that medication is not needed or not effective Presence of health issues such as poor vision or arthritis

Related to health condition	Health condition has no symptoms (lack of cues that drug therapy is needed), such as high cholesterol, osteoporosis Chronic condition that needs long-term treatment Health condition is associated with a stigma, such as depression or dementia
Related to medication	Adverse drug reactions Administration technique that requires special knowledge to use correctly; for example, use of inhalers, eye drops, or an injectable medication Complex regimens—for example, must be taken multiple times per day or at a specific time of day
Related to finances	High cost of the medication High co-pay for a physician visit Drug not covered by insurance
Related to health-care system	Poor communication with physician Multiple providers involved in care Difficulty accessing physician or pharmacy

Too often medication adherence is viewed as a problem that rests solely with the patient. However, nonadherence is impacted by multiple factors as reflected by the five categories of barriers. The patient-specific factor is only one of them. Indeed, nonadherence needs to be recognized as a complex problem, for which the solution requires a joint effort between patients and multiple members of the health-care team who can support the patient and family members as needed. Pharmacists have extensive knowledge about adherence barriers and strategies to address poor adherence and are a key resource on the health-care team. As an aside, occupational therapists are an underappreciated but valuable resource to assist with medication adherence efforts.[233]

Regardless of what external barriers might be present, the crux of medication adherence is that ultimately it is a behavior, similar to other health behaviors. As with the examples of exercising regularly and eating vegetables, making adherence part of a daily routine is easier said than done for many people. What influences a person's ability or willingness to take on the behavior of being adherent with their medications?

The World Health Organization (WHO) emphasizes that both motivation and information (about the medication and illness) are necessary to lead to a change in behavior.[234] In this case, the behavior is improved adherence. From other research, we have learned that patient beliefs play an important role. Three beliefs that influence adherence are the patient's belief that (1) the medication is necessary, (2) its benefits are greater than potential safety concerns, and (3) the medication is affordable.[235] Coincidentally, these beliefs mirror the reasons already listed that older adults cite for not adhering.

Ultimately, each person's situation is unique. Individuals can experience myriad combinations of adherence barriers. There is neither a one-size-fits-all solution nor a formula for how to "fix" adherence issues, which makes tackling the problem of adherence so challenging. Uncovering barriers requires conversations that explore each patient's medication-related beliefs and experiences. Often a patient's caregivers, friends, and family can play an important supportive role and should be included in problem-solving. Joint efforts to address barriers are key. It clearly is a team endeavor, with the patient being the center of that team.

PATIENT ROLE IN ADDRESSING NONADHERENCE

Good medication adherence is a tool that empowers patients to manage their chronic health conditions. Viewed in this light, awareness of issues surrounding medication adherence—or nonadherence—enables you to become more engaged in drug therapy decisions and in turn achieve better control of your health. Your physicians may not share your same perspective or priorities regarding drug therapy. Thus, you need to speak up about what matters most to you. As an informed patient, ask to be part of drug-therapy decisions, because ultimately, it is you who will be taking those medications at home. Get a family member involved to support your medication adherence. The more eyes and ears that can help you understand your medications and health conditions, the more you'll feel encouraged and motivated to follow through. Sometimes a prompt or reminder is all that is needed. If you find that you tend to miss more than an occasional dose of a medication, reach out to a member of your health-care team or family to find ways to address what is getting in your way.

Education and information are power when it comes to adherence. Seek information from your pharmacist with each new medication. Talk about the medication instructions and make sure you understand them. Pharmacists are excellent resources to educate you about your medications and help reduce adherence barriers. Patients who have sufficient information about their medications generally have better adherence.[236] Request an annual medication review to identify and eliminate unnecessary or potentially harmful medicines. In this way, you can focus on having better adherence to a smaller number of medications that are truly necessary and beneficial.

The responsibility of taking your medications ultimately falls on you, as the patient, but you should not feel alone in the process. Most patients do not talk about adherence issues unless they are asked. However, when was the last time a physician asked if you had any problems with taking your medications or in getting them refilled? The topic continues to remain outside the realm of a routine office visit. Physicians might not bring up adherence for different reasons. Some still view it as a problem solely for the patient. Others recognize that it is a hard topic to ask about and get an honest answer from patients, for reasons discussed earlier. Thus, the most important take-home messages here are (1) bring up medication adherence with your health-care team and (2) be honest when asked. One of my clients illustrates problems that can arise when you are not proactive about medication concerns.

At age sixty-six, Candace was prescribed amlodipine to manage her blood pressure. She took it on most days of the week, but forgot it if she had her grandchildren overnight or had to leave the house early to get to an activity. Three months later, Candace's blood pressure was improved but still above the goal of 130/80 mmHg. Her physician increased the dose of amlodipine. Candace started taking the higher dose but noticed she was urinating more often and had swelling in her ankles. Bothered by these side effects, she reduced amlodipine to every other day, which made the side effects more tolerable. Six months later at her doctor's office, Candace's blood pressure was still high, so the doctor added a new blood pressure medicine, enalapril. Candace filled the enalapril prescription but took it on days opposite her amlodipine because she was concerned about side effects. The next time Candace saw her physician, her blood pressure had barely improved. The doctor this time added the diuretic hydrochlorothiazide to her regimen, determined to reach Candace's blood pressure goal. By the time I met with Candace, she was prescribed three blood pressure medications and not fully adherent to any of them. Once I uncovered the adherence issues, I brought them to the attention of her physician who promptly adjusted her blood pressure medicines and helped Candace understand the importance of adherence and communicating with her physician in the future.

Candace never spoke up about how she took her medicines at home or voiced her concerns about side effects. On the other hand, Candace's physician never asked and incorrectly assumed she was taking her medications as instructed. If only Candace had spoken up or her physician had confirmed Candace's adherence, how different the story would have unfolded. The lesson here is to recognize the role of nonadherence and the importance of talking about it, even if you have to bring it up. If your health-care provider does ask how often you miss doses of your medications, be honest. You might be surprised to learn that physicians will be grateful to know the truth, as it will make their jobs easier. Similarly, pharmacists know how hard it can be to take multiple medications daily, so when we ask, take advantage of the question, knowing how important the discussion can be. Voicing your beliefs and attitudes about medications with your health-care team is part of the process of providing person-centered care and care that aligns with what matters most to you.

SUMMARY

Medication adherence is not routinely talked about during routine office visits, yet it is paramount to good health outcomes. It is defined as the extent to which individuals take their medications as instructed. Nonadherence is considered a preventable medication-related problem, which means individuals have the opportunity to improve adherence to achieve better health outcomes. Importantly, nonadherence is common and typically caused by more than one barrier. Identifying and addressing barriers is not just the responsibility of the patient, but often requires involvement of other members of the health-care team. Pharmacists are excellent resources to help individuals achieve better adherence.

Understanding the concept of medication adherence allows individuals to be more proactive to bring up questions or concerns about their medications and how to take them correctly. This chapter provides space for individuals to consider their own adherence patterns without feeling embarrassed if those patterns are less than ideal. Chapter 17 continues this conversation with specific tips and strategies to improve adherence.

KEY POINTS

- Medication adherence is defined as the extent to which a patient correctly follows medication instructions.
- Nonadherence is a common preventable medication-related problem. It is caused by myriad factors that are unique to each person and can be intentional or unintentional.
- There is no single approach to improve adherence. Efforts must be tailored to each person's situation and require a joint effort between the individual and the health-care team.
- Steps individuals can take to improve adherence include being honest about how often they miss doses of their medications and making sure they understand basic information about their medications and health conditions.

Chapter 9

Understanding Drug Interactions

One of the most common concerns patients have when they request a medication review is about whether their medications "mix well" together. In other words, do their medications interact? Drug interaction indeed is an important topic. Yet, at the same time, it is complicated to discuss because there are many variables that can impact whether or not an interaction will lead to a meaningful issue for an individual. Some interactions are clinically important and require adjustment to the medications to avoid an adverse event. Others may have no noticeable effect and therefore no adjustments are needed.

Older adults are at high risk of experiencing a drug interaction because they frequently take multiple medications and have multiple chronic health conditions. This means there are more chances for a drug to interact. Interactions are more challenging to predict, detect, and manage in older adults because every individual has a unique situation. Symptoms that result from a drug interaction can mimic another medical problem. If the drug interaction is not detected as the cause of those symptoms, it can lead to additional medications being prescribed.

As discussed in Chapter 3, drug interactions are one of the eight categories of medication-related problems (MRPs) and often can be prevented. Thus, this topic is relevant when it comes to improving safe medication use, as many harmful drug interactions can be avoided when individuals are more engaged with their drug therapy and informed about important interactions. This chapter explains the nature of drug interactions and different factors that impact the chance of a harmful interaction. It also provides information to empower individuals to ask questions and be proactive to prevent a serious problem from developing.

DRUG INTERACTIONS DEFINED

A drug interaction is a change or alteration in the way a drug acts in the body that is caused by another drug, food, alcohol, or nutrients and dietary supplements. Drugs also can interact with or alter a disease state (health condition), typically leading to a worsening of the condition. When asking about "drug interactions," most people have in mind reactions between two or more drugs; however, other types of drug interactions are equally important and can lead to significant problems under the right circumstances. Drugs interacting with disease states are possibly more common than drug-drug interactions. Drug-disease interactions can be an important source of negative health outcomes in older adults. The five categories of drug interactions are summarized in **Table 9-1** with examples of each. Note that this table contains only a few examples to illustrate each type of interaction and is not a complete listing. Each category is explained in more detail in the next section. Interactions with cannabis, or marijuana, also are addressed briefly. Recommendations about seeking drug interaction information on the internet are provided in Chapter 19.

Table 9.1 Drug Interaction Categories

Drug interaction category	Examples of interacting combinations	Clinical effect
Drug-drug interactions	Verapamil added to simvastatin or amlodipine added to simvastatin	Decreased metabolism of simvastatin leading to increased simvastatin levels and risk of adverse effects

	Gabapentin combined with oxycodone or another opioid pain medicine	Increased the risk of severe sedation and slowed breathing (enhanced drug side effects)
	Carbamazepine added to verapamil	Increased metabolism of verapamil and decreased effectiveness
Drug-disease interactions	NSAIDs and high blood pressure (hypertension)	Increased blood pressure
	Amitriptyline, diphenhydramine, oxybutynin (plus other drugs with anticholinergic properties*) and dementia or mild cognitive impairment	Increased risk of confusion, worsened cognitive function
	NSAIDs or antacids with high sodium content and heart failure	Increased fluid retention and worsened heart failure symptoms
Drug-food interactions	High-protein meals and levodopa/carbidopa	Decreased absorption of levodopa/carbidopa; delayed onset of effect
	Grapefruit juice and verapamil, diltiazem, amlodipine, and felodipine (as well as many other drugs)	Increased absorption leading to increased clinical and adverse effects
	Green leafy vegetables and other foods that are high in vitamin K and warfarin	Vitamin K decreases effectiveness of warfarin

Drug-nutrient or supplement interactions	Calcium or iron products combined with levothyroxine	Decreased absorption of levothyroxine when taken at the same time
	Ginseng, gingko or garlic combined with warfarin, clopidogrel, or aspirin	Increased risk of bleeding
	Vitamin B$_{12}$ and long-term use of metformin	Decreased vitamin B$_{12}$ levels
Drug-alcohol interactions	Alprazolam, diazepam, lorazepam, zolpidem and other sedative-hypnotic drugs and alcohol	Increased sedation and fall risk
	Warfarin and alcohol	Short-term heavy alcohol intake increases warfarin levels and bleeding risk; chronic alcohol use increases metabolism and decreases effectiveness of warfarin
	Acetaminophen and alcohol	Increased risk of liver damage

*Drugs with anticholinergic properties are discussed in more detail in Chapters 9 and 10.

NSAIDs = Nonsteroidal anti-inflammatory drugs

There are two major mechanisms of how drug interactions occur that are worth briefly defining. The mechanism of a drug interaction is relevant because it determines how we manage different interactions. The first mechanism is an interaction that alters how a drug is absorbed, metabolized, or eliminated. You might recognize these as pharmacokinetic parameters described in Chapter 2. Pharmacokinetic-type interactions can cause either an increase or decrease in the amount of drug in the body, depending on the nature of the interaction. If it leads to increased levels, then greater-than-expected effects are anticipated, which can mean a greater clinical effect and/or exaggerated adverse drug reaction. If it leads to decreased levels in the body, the result can be reduced effectiveness of the medication and failure to manage the health condition. Either result can be clinically important and might require adjustments to the medication combination. Drug interactions that increase or decrease the metabolism of other drugs are among the most common and well-documented interactions.

Calcium is an example of a drug—or more specifically a supplement—that can reduce the absorption of other drugs from the intestinal tract. For example, calcium should not be taken at the same time as levothyroxine because of this interaction. Verapamil illustrates a metabolism-based interaction. Verapamil treats blood pressure and heart rhythm problems; however, it also slows the metabolism of simvastatin, a drug that lowers cholesterol levels. Because simvastatin's metabolism is slowed, it causes higher concentrations of simvastatin in the body and thus increased side effects. Options to manage this interaction include lowering the dose of simvastatin or avoiding the combination altogether. Finally, lithium illustrates an elimination-based interaction. Lithium treats bipolar depression and is eliminated from the body via the kidneys. Losartan is a blood pressure medicine that can slow or reduce the ability of lithium to reach the kidney where it ultimately is removed from the body. This results in higher lithium concentrations in the bloodstream and potential toxicity. The interaction requires careful monitoring of lithium blood levels or avoiding the combination in some cases.

The other major mechanism for drug interactions is an interaction that alters the effect the drug has on the body. This is a pharmacodynamic type of interaction. This type of interaction can lead to an additive effect of the drug on the body (and thus increased clinical or adverse effects) or the interacting drugs can oppose each other in the body, essentially countering the effectiveness of either drug. An example of an additive effect is when warfarin, a drug that is used to prevent blood clots and can increase the risk of bleeding, is combined with ibuprofen, an anti-inflammatory pain medicine that also can increase bleeding. This leads to an interaction in which there is an exaggerated effect, namely greater risk of bleeding. In contrast, an example of an interaction where two drugs counter the effect of each other is when donepezil, a drug to treat Alzheimer's dementia, is combined with oxybutynin, a drug to treat overactive bladder. Donepezil works by activating certain nerve receptors in the brain, while oxybutynin works by blocking these same nerve receptors. Thus, each drug opposes the effect of the other, leading to decreased effectiveness of both drugs.

CATEGORIES OF DRUG INTERACTIONS

By far, drug-drug interactions are the most well-studied and receive the most attention when individuals think about drug interactions. Every drug approved by the FDA must undergo research to evaluate drug interactions. This means that clinicians have a good sense of the drug-drug interaction potential for prescription drugs. A few examples are provided in **Table 9-1**. Fortunately, most medications have a wide window of safety, so minor interactions that lead to small increases or decreases in the concentration of a drug are clinically unimportant. However, there are several interactions that are considered significant enough that intervention is warranted to avoid an adverse drug reaction. It is beyond the scope of this book to list them all here. Suffice it to know that these interactions are well-documented and thus easily identified. For these medications, it is important to anticipate the interaction and adjust drug therapy to prevent harm. A handful of drug-drug interactions has been identified as a particular concern in older adults because the interactions have been associated with increased risk of harm, including hospitalization. They are listed in **Table 9-2**. These combinations need to be approached with caution or avoided when possible.[237,238]

Table 9-2. Serious Drug-Drug Interactions in Older Adults

Object drug or drug class	Interacting drugs or drug class	Reaction
Angiotensin converting enzyme (ACE) inhibitors (such as enalapril, lisinopril); angiotensin receptor blockers (such as losartan, valsartan)	Amiloride, eplerenone, spironolactone, triamterene (a subset of diuretics or water pills)	Increased risk of high potassium levels
Lithium	ACE inhibitors, bumetanide, furosemide	Increased lithium levels and risk of lithium toxicity
Opioid pain medicines (such as hydrocodone, morphine, oxycodone)	Benzodiazepines (such as alprazolam, diazepam, lorazepam)	Increased risk of opioid overdose, slowed breathing, excess sedation
Opioid pain medicines	Gabapentin, pregabalin	Increased risk of severe sedation and slowed breathing
Warfarin	Amiodarone, NSAIDs (such as ibuprofen, naproxen)	Increased risk of bleeding
Warfarin	Certain antibiotics: clarithromycin, erythromycin, ciprofloxacin, trimethoprim/sulfamethoxazole (TMP/SMX, Bactrim, Septra)	Increased risk of bleeding

NSAIDs = nonsteroidal anti-inflammatory drugs

Drug-disease interactions are unique among the interaction categories listed in **Table 9-1** because with drug-disease interactions, the effect is on a health condition, rather than another medication. Drug-disease interactions are estimated to occur in 20 percent of older adults and are thought to be more common than drug-drug interactions.[239] Unfortunately, potential for a drug to interact with one's health conditions often is overlooked. Common examples of drug-disease interactions are also listed in **Table 9-1**. Drug-disease interactions that involve over-the-counter (OTC) products also are very important to be aware of. Warnings about interactions with health conditions must be included on OTC drug labels; however, the wording sometimes is vague and unclear to consumers.[240] Thus, the expertise of a pharmacist can be very valuable to double check for relevant interactions when choosing nonprescription products.

Drug-food interactions are another type of drug interaction. Food can affect the ability or extent of a drug to be absorbed from the intestinal tract into blood circulation. Often, this interaction is used in a positive way to reduce side effects. For example, the blood pressure and heart medication carvedilol is recommended to be taken with food to slow its absorption and reduce the risk of a sharp reduction in blood pressure. Other drug-food interactions are more specific; for example, grapefruit affects metabolism of many drugs, resulting in increased levels of the medications and increased side effects. Other examples are found in **Table 9-1**. To manage drug-food interactions, medications might have specific instructions, such as to take with food or on an empty stomach. Other interactions are managed by limiting or avoiding certain types of foods. Bottom-line, it is important to pay attention to warnings about drug-food interactions and heed instructions so that you take medications safely with regard to meals or food restrictions. When in doubt, do not guess; check with your pharmacist.

The next category of interactions is with specific nutrients and dietary supplements. Recall from Chapter 6 that dietary supplements behave like medications and can contribute to interactions. As with other types of interactions, nutrient- and dietary supplement–interactions can result in decreased or increased effects of a prescribed medication. Calcium and iron are known to block the absorption of certain medications, reducing drug effectiveness. The reverse also happens, in that medications can impact the level of nutrients in the body. For example, long-term use of metformin (a diabetes medicine) can lead to low levels of vitamin B_{12}, and long-term use of omeprazole (a drug that reduces production of stomach acid) can lead to decreased magnesium levels. Diuretics (water pills) can cause decreased levels of potassium and magnesium in the body, while a subset of diuretics can increase calcium levels. These and other nutrient interactions that are well-known can be watched for to avoid a problem from developing. It is important that you never stop taking a medication out of concern about an interaction. Always discuss with your physician or pharmacist first.

Drug-alcohol interactions are important to recognize because (a) alcohol can interact with many medications and disease states, and (b) alcohol use is not always discussed between patients and their healthcare team. It can be sensitive subject, and some patients may not fully disclose how much alcohol they drink. Many people might think their alcohol use doesn't impact their health. However, there can be important consequences if not included when talking about drug interactions. For example, alcohol can increase the risk of bleeding with warfarin, aspirin, and nonsteroidal anti-inflammatory drugs (NSAIDs); it can exacerbate the sedating side effects of medications and increase the risk of a fall; and alcohol can make it more difficult to manage hypertension, diabetes, gout, and insomnia.[241]

Another source of drug interactions that is of emerging significance is with cannabis, also known as marijuana. The majority of states in the United States now have legalized cannabis for medical or recreational use. There are numerous active substances within the cannabis plant. The most well-known are cannabidiol (CBD) and delta-9-tetrahydrocannabinol (THC). CBD and other cannabis-derived products are increasingly used by older adults. These products carry the potential for significant interactions with prescribed medications and health conditions.[242] It is extremely important therefore to include cannabis in a drug interaction review. Do not assume that the cannabis dispensary did such a review for you. Ask for a review from your pharmacist and be sure he or she knows what cannabis products you take.

PREVENTING, PREDICTING, AND MANAGING DRUG INTERACTIONS

Drug interactions are estimated to occur in 35 to 60 percent of older adults and are more likely as the number of medications increases.[243,244,245] However only a fraction of drug interactions result in a clinically important adverse drug event. Most severe, potentially harmful interactions are well-known. Ideally, we can prevent serious interactions before harm occurs.

To protect consumers, safeguards are built into the medication use process. Software programs that screen for drug interactions are designed to alert prescribers and pharmacists to serious drug-drug interactions so corrections can be made before the medication reaches the patient. These software programs are extremely valuable but also have limitations. Any screening program can only screen for the medications that are on record for a patient. Thus, nonprescription products, drug samples from a doctor's office, or prescriptions filled at a different pharmacy cannot be evaluated. Additionally, the programs generally evaluate only drug-drug interactions and won't capture drug-disease interactions, for example.

Another safeguard against serious interactions is the consumer information that is provided with each medication dispensed at the pharmacy. This written material is designed for the patient and includes information on drug interactions. The material can be hard to read and may not be complete, but it still offers important information.[246] Ideally, it is best to speak one-on-one with your pharmacist to get information about interactions when starting a new medication.

Many interactions are well-known and the decision of how to handle them is clear. Minor interactions are considered low risk and no action is needed. Major interactions are most serious and typically need to be avoided by switching to different medications or reducing drug doses.

For example, when simvastatin and verapamil are used together, the dose of simvastatin needs to be reduced. Most interactions fall somewhere in between and are considered to be potentially important. For these interactions, clinicians must use their expertise and experience to predict if an interaction will be clinically meaningful for an individual.

Predicting whether an interaction will be clinically meaningful, however, gets complicated and cannot always be done with certainty. Each person has a unique medication list, health conditions, and kidney and liver function. In addition, drug-specific details need to be factored in, such as the drug dose and route of administration, as well as a person's age, overall health, and nutritional status. An important interaction for one person might not cause a problem for someone else. Physicians and pharmacists often work together to determine the best approach, with input from patients on their preferences and what matters most to them.

For interactions where the impact for a particular person is uncertain, the best option often is to educate the patient about the interaction, what symptoms to look for, and what actions to take if symptoms occur. If the interaction has to do with one drug affecting the absorption of another drug, it might be possible to separate when the two drugs are taken to avoid the problem. For other major interactions, a drug might need to be switched to one that does not interact.

Sometimes a drug interaction can be managed by creating what is called a "stable interaction." This means that two interacting drugs can be used safely together as long as the dosages of the drugs are adjusted to account for the interaction. It is important to note, though, that if one drug of a stable interaction is removed, it will throw the remaining drug off balance. The dose of the remaining drug would then need to be adjusted. This is another important reason why you should never stop taking a medication without first checking with your pharmacist or physician. Similarly, if you are aware of a drug interaction on your medication list, do not make changes on your own. Always confer with your pharmacist or physician.

One last topic to include for completeness is the role of pharmacogenomics in helping to predict drug interactions. Pharmacogenomics is the study of how genes in our DNA affect the body's response to certain medications. This information helps personalize drug therapy selection to improve effectiveness and reduce harm. An individual's pharmacogenomic test results provide information on how a person metabolizes specific drugs. This information enables clinicians to anticipate drug interactions that will be clinically important for an individual and to take action to manage or avoid them.

The science of pharmacogenomics is fairly new. Pharmacogenomic testing is in its early stages, with a growing appreciation of the value it brings to patient care. However, it is not yet widely adopted as part of routine practice, nor is testing universally covered by insurance. Our understanding of pharmacogenomics and how to integrate this information into the health-care process will continue to evolve in the coming years. It is anticipated that pharmacogenomic testing will become a mainstream part of care as another tool to guide drug therapy selection.

HOW TO REDUCE THE RISK OF DRUG INTERACTIONS

Older adults are at increased risk of drug interactions for a variety of reasons: polypharmacy, involvement of multiple prescribers, and age-related changes in how the body handles medications and how drugs affect the body. In addition, older adults have multiple chronic health conditions, which increase the potential for a drug-disease interaction. There is much variability patient-to-patient, which can make it difficult to predict the impact of an interaction for a specific person. Interactions in an older patient can be harder to detect because the symptoms might be nonspecific and not recognized as being drug-induced. A person might have symptoms of low blood pressure, confusion, or feeling tired or weak, or perhaps they had a fall. The physician might attribute the cause to another medical condition and not suspect an interaction, thus delaying the ability to correct the problem.

Knowing that many serious drug interactions can be prevented, what can patients do—what can *you* do—to become more involved in the process and reduce the risk of a serious problem?

- Strive to use one pharmacy for all of your medications so that the pharmacist can screen for interactions. Note that community pharmacists will not know about medications filled at a different pharmacy (including mail order), nonprescription medications you take, and medication samples from your doctor unless you provide this information.
- Bring a complete list of your medications to each health-care encounter so that the pharmacist or physician can review all of the medicines you take. The list needs to include OTC drugs and dietary supplements.
- Read labels of your OTC products and the warning labels added to your prescription medication bottles. This is where you can find warnings about interactions with drugs, medical conditions, food, and alcohol.
- Ask questions about drug interactions. Recognize that drugs interact with more than just other drugs. Be sure you know about food interactions, and also those with alcohol or cannabis, if these apply to you. Check with a pharmacist when choosing an OTC product or dietary supplement. Finally, ask about the possibility of interactions any time a new medication is added or stopped (in case it can destabilize a stable interaction).
- If you are taking medications that have the potential for a low-risk interaction (not serious enough to warrant changing therapy), make sure you are informed of what symptoms to be on the lookout for; be part of the plan to detect a potential problem early.

- If you notice a new symptom that is troublesome, check with your pharmacist or physician in case it could be the result of a drug interaction; maybe it's your medications.

A final comment is to remember the importance of taking only the medications that are of true benefit to your health. Continuing to take medications that no longer are needed or helpful can increase the chance of an interaction. Therefore, work closely with your physician and pharmacist to identify opportunities to safely reduce medications when possible. Never stop taking medications on your own. Chapter 16 addresses strategies to decrease unnecessary medication use.

SUMMARY

Drug interactions comprise a complex topic that encompasses interaction between not just other medications, but also between health conditions, food, nutrients, and alcohol. Interactions with medical marijuana also need to be considered. Older adults are at increased risk of experiencing adverse events as a result of these interactions, which makes prevention key. While safeguards are in place in our drug distribution system to catch and prevent many interactions before they reach the patient, the safeguards are not foolproof. Thus, patient involvement remains an important part of efforts to avoid serious interactions.

Minimizing the risk of clinically meaningful drug interactions requires patients to be knowledgeable about their medications and to know to ask questions about interactions. A greater awareness of the importance of drug interactions empowers patients to be proactive with their health-care team and in their own home to reduce the risk of this common medication-related problem.

KEY POINTS

- The topic of drug interactions is complex and involves interactions between drugs and other drugs, as well as with medical conditions, food, nutrients, and alcohol.
- Many drug interactions are not clinically important; others are known to be associated with harm in older adults.
- There is much variability person-to-person, which limits the ability to predict with certainty whether some interaction will be clinically important for a person.
- Patients can proactively reduce the risk of serious drug interactions by inquiring about interactions when medications are added or stopped and when selecting nonprescription products for self-care.
- When new symptoms appear, it best to err on the safe side and suspect it could be the medications. Check with your physician or pharmacist.

Chapter 10

Potentially Inappropriate Medications for Older Adults

All medications have clinical benefits that need to be balanced against their potential for harm. This is particularly true for older adults who are at increased risk of experiencing problems. Fortunately, the desirable effects of the majority of medications far outweigh the chance of serious problems. Age can affect this balance, however, mostly as a result of changes in how the body handles and responds to medications. These are the pharmacokinetic and pharmacodynamic changes described in Chapter 2. The good news is that only certain medications are identified as being somewhat riskier as we get older. These medications are the focus of this and the next chapter. Furthermore, many of the adverse effects are preventable. Knowledge and awareness are key. Informed patients and family members play an important role in working with their clinicians to identify when these medications are necessary and appropriate to be prescribed, and when safer options can be used instead.

This chapter focuses on medications that have been identified by geriatrics experts as being potentially inappropriate in older individuals. The term "potentially inappropriate medications" (PIMs) refers to specific drugs for which the potential for adverse effects is thought to be greater than the clinical benefits. Selection of an improper drug was introduced in Chapter 3 as one of the eight categories of MRPs. PIMs fall into this category, thus making it an important topic as we discuss safe medication use.

At the same time, patients and consumers are not expected to have the expertise when it comes to drug selection. They naturally rely on their prescribers. You might ask, "What good is this information to patients if they don't have a medical or pharmacy degree?" Granted, the material about PIMs and high-risk medications might be difficult to fully understand, as it is about specific medications and their effects on the body. Rest assured the medications mentioned here indeed can be used without problem for many individuals. The purpose of this and the next chapter is to inform older adults and family members more broadly that there are medications that should be used with greater care—some should be avoided and some should be used with more caution. I cannot say what your situation is, but if you see a medication here that you or a loved one are taking, discuss it with your health-care team. Do not apply this information on your own and never stop a medication without first talking with your physician or pharmacist.

OVERVIEW OF POTENTIALLY INAPPROPRIATE MEDICATION USE

PIM use is associated with preventable medication-related problems such as adverse drug reactions and drug interactions and is associated with increased use of health-care services such as extra outpatient visits, emergency department visits, and hospitalizations.[247] It is estimated that 34 percent of older adults are prescribed at least one PIM.[248] The good news is that the frequency of PIM use among older adults has gradually been declining over time[249] as a result of greater awareness about PIMs and efforts to reduce inappropriate prescribing. This trend is good, but there is still room for improvement. Research published in the *Journal of the American Geriatrics Society* estimated that 7.3 billion doses of PIMs were dispensed in 2018, corresponding to $4.4 billion in spending.[250]

DEFINING POTENTIALLY INAPPROPRIATE MEDICATIONS

A PIM is a medication for which the potential for adverse effects is thought to be greater than the clinical benefits, especially when there are safer or more effective choices available. Experts recommend that health professionals and patients discuss these medications when it comes to therapy options because they may not be the safest or most effective choices for older individuals in certain situations. For many of these PIMs, there are safer options available that can be used instead. It is important to understand that these medications are *potentially* inappropriate, not *definitely* inappropriate for older individuals. This distinction is critical: there are many examples of when a drug identified as a PIM is a reasonable option for an individual. Patients should never make changes to their drug therapy without talking with their physician or pharmacist first. The information in this chapter helps to open the door for these conversations.

In 1991, the first "official" list of PIMs was published in the medical literature.[251] I was a new pharmacist at the time and recall the momentous nature of that article. It was the first time that anyone had compiled a list that explicitly defined high risk medications. Importantly, it elevated the awareness that certain medications may not be the best choice in older individuals. The geriatrician Dr. Mark Beers authored this initial publication, and the PIM list came to be called the Beers Criteria. Since 1991, it has undergone several updates and revisions. Today it remains one of the most highly regarded PIM lists, as discussed in the next section.

The process of defining specific drugs as PIMs has evolved over the last thirty years. Early versions of the Beers Criteria were based on consensus among geriatrics experts because there was very little research available in older adults. Today, expert consensus is still an important part of the process, but the experts have much more research on which to base their decisions, making these criteria even more robust.

EXPERT LISTINGS OF POTENTIALLY INAPPROPRIATE MEDICATIONS

Several expert listings that identify PIMs have been developed internationally over the years, which signals a universal priority to improve the quality of prescribing in the older population. The two most recognized lists are described in this section, along with discussion of some of the specific medications or groups of medications that are considered potentially inappropriate.

The first is the American Geriatrics Society's (AGS) Beers Criteria, which was developed in the United States in 1991, as mentioned.[252] The original AGS Beers Criteria were developed for nursing home residents.[253] Health professionals quickly realized these criteria also could apply beyond the nursing home setting. Thus, over the years, the Beers Criteria have undergone extensive revisions and expansion and now apply to nearly all older adults, regardless of where they reside.[254] Following the death of Dr. Beers, the responsibility of updating the criteria was taken on by the AGS and the name officially changed to AGS Beers. Regular updates are scheduled every three years. The most recent update was published in May 2023. It includes over two dozen high risk medications plus a list of drugs that are potentially inappropriate when used in patients with certain health conditions or syndromes, such as heart failure and cognitive impairment, or who are a high fall risk. In addition, it includes a list of medications to be used with caution, a list of significant interactions, and selected medications that need to be used at lower doses or with caution in patients with reduced kidney function.

The second well-respected listing is a pair of criteria known by the acronym STOPP/START, which were developed in Europe in 2008.[255] The acronym STOPP stands for Screening Tool of Older People's Prescriptions, while START stands for Screening Tool to Alert to Right Treatment. The START criteria address inappropriate medication use from the perspective of medications that are not prescribed for a patient but should be. It is discussed separately in Chapter 12.

The STOPP list was revised in 2015 and contains eighty criteria that define specific situations where certain medications are high-risk and should be avoided in older adults. The STOPP list is unique because it includes three noteworthy criteria that are not specific to any particular drug or drug class but are central to good medication management in older adults:

1. Every medication should have an "evidence-based clinical indication." Worded another way, every medication should have a current, valid clinical reason for why it is prescribed.

2. Medications should not be used "beyond the recommended duration," when the duration for the drug is well-defined. This statement refers to the importance of not continuing medications long-term unless there is a clear reason to do so. This criterion draws attention to medications that are renewed and continued but might not be needed any longer, otherwise known as "prescribing inertia."

3. An individual should not take two medications from the same drug class. A drug class refers to a group of drugs that are closely related either by chemical structure or the way they work in the body. Drugs that work in the same way in the body generally do not offer additional benefit if used in combination but can increase the risk of side effects. An example of duplicate medications is a person who is prescribed two blood pressure medications that are both from the beta-blocker drug class, like metoprolol and atenolol, or someone taking both ibuprofen and naproxen, which are both non-steroidal anti-inflammatory drugs (NSAIDs).

These three STOPP criteria are of universal value to anyone who takes medications and should be part of every medication review. A study that evaluated drug regimens of over seven hundred hospitalized older adults found that one-third (34 percent) of these patients did not have a current, valid reason documented for their medications.[256] Remember, too, that these three criteria apply to all medications a person takes, including over-the-counter (OTC) drugs and dietary supplements that were the focus of Chapter 6.

Tables 10-1 and 10-2 provide examples of PIMs from AGS Beers Criteria and STOPP. To help you understand the value of these PIM listings, six groups of drugs common to both sets of criteria are described in the next list. These reflect medications that are commonly used but warrant extra care when prescribed in older adults. It deserves repeating that PIMs are *potentially* inappropriate, not *definitely*. Each person has a unique situation. This information explains the possible risks surrounding these medications and ideally can be used to start the conversations between individuals and their health-care team.

Table 10-1. Examples of Potentially Inappropriate Medication Criteria in AGS Beers Criteria

Medication/condition	Recommendation	Reason
Potentially inappropriate medication use		
Antihistamines such as diphenhydramine, meclizine, hydroxyzine, others	Avoid	Highly anticholinergic; risk of confusion, dry mouth, constipation, among other effects
Antipsychotic drugs to treat behavioral symptoms of dementia or for "as needed" use with dementia or cognitive impairment	Avoid—with exceptions for treating schizophrenia or bipolar disease	Can increase the risk of stroke or even death; increased fall risk
Aspirin for preventing a first heart attack or stroke	Do not start aspirin in patients who have never had a heart attack or stroke	Risk of major bleeding increases with older age

Benzodiazepines	Avoid (certain exceptions are specified)	Increased sensitivity to adverse effects; risk of cognitive impairment, falls, fractures
Chlorpropamide, glimepiride, glyburide (specific diabetes drugs only)	Avoid	Higher risk of prolonged low blood sugar levels (hypoglycemia)
Digoxin	Should not be the first-choice drug for treating heart failure or irregular heart rhythm because safer options are available	Risk of toxicity in patients with reduced kidney function; lower dose is needed
Muscle relaxants, such as carisoprodol, cyclobenzaprine, methocarbamol, others	Avoid	Most of these drugs are poorly tolerated, and older adults unable to take effective dose; sedation, fall, and fracture risk
Nonsteroidal anti-inflammatory drugs (NSAIDs)	Avoid long-term use unless other options are not available; use with caution if kidney problems or heart failure	Risk of bleeding, can increase blood pressure; can worsen heart failure

Potentially inappropriate medications because of interaction with a health condition		
Dementia or cognitive impairment	Avoid anticholinergic drugs, BZDs, and non-BZDs (sleep medicines)	Can increase risk of confusion, falls
Heart failure, moderate to severe symptoms	Avoid diltiazem or verapamil	Risk of worsening heart failure symptoms
Urinary incontinence in women	Avoid doxazosin, prazosin, and terazosin	Can worsen incontinence

BZD = benzodiazepine

Table 10-2. Examples of Potentially Inappropriate Medications from STOPP Criteria

Category	Sample criteria that describe when the medications are potentially inappropriate
Cardiovascular system	• Verapamil or diltiazem in patients who have moderate to severe symptoms of heart failure, because these drugs may worsen heart failure
Antiplatelet/ anticoagulant drugs	• Long-term aspirin at doses greater than 160 mg per day, because of increased bleeding and no evidence of greater effectiveness • NSAIDs and anticoagulant drugs used in combination, because of increased risk of gastrointestinal bleeding

Central nervous system and psychotropic drugs	• Anticholinergic drugs in patients who have delirium or dementia, because these drugs can worsen cognitive impairment • Older antihistamines, such as chlorpheniramine, diphenhydramine, and doxylamine; because safer, less harmful antihistamines are now available
Musculoskeletal system	• NSAIDs in patients with severe hypertension or severe heart failure, because NSAIDs can worsen either condition
Endocrine system	• Beta-blockers (such as atenolol, carvedilol, and metoprolol, among others) in patients with diabetes who have frequent episodes of low blood sugar, because beta-blockers can mask most symptoms of low blood sugar
Drugs that predictably increase the risk of falls in older people	• Benzodiazepines, because they are sedating and can impair balance

NSAID = nonsteroidal anti-inflammatory drug; PPI = proton pump inhibitor

- **Drugs with strong anticholinergic effects.** Anticholinergic effects are explained in more detail in the next chapter; however, a brief description here is warranted. Anticholinergic drugs are associated with troublesome adverse effects in older patients such as dry mouth, constipation, blurred vision, sedation, and confusion. Of particular concern in older adults is the association with cognitive impairment, namely, decreased memory, confusion, dementia, and delirium.[257] Safer options and nondrug therapy are preferred. It is important to note that many OTC antihistamines, such as diphenhydramine, chlorpheniramine, and doxylamine, are strong anticholinergic drugs. These drugs are older allergy medications (called "first-generation antihistamines"), but they often are ingredients in cough and cold products and sleep products. In general, newer antihistamines are safer and more appropriate choices for older adults.

The impact of anticholinergic drugs on cognitive function is additive, meaning that the greater amount of these types of drugs a person is taking, the greater the risk. Thus, a good medication review with someone who has the expertise to identify drugs that have anticholinergic properties is essential.

- **Use of benzodiazepines (BZDs; to treat anxiety or insomnia) and nonbenzodiazepines (non-BZDs; to treat insomnia).** There are several BZDs approved to treat anxiety or insomnia; common examples include alprazolam (Xanax®), clonazepam (Klonopin®), diazepam (Valium®), and temazepam (Restoril®). Non-BZDs are approved only to treat insomnia and include eszopiclone (Lunesta®), zaleplon (Sonata®), and zolpidem (Ambien®).

  BZDs and non-BZDs are associated with serious adverse effects like confusion, sedation, impaired balance, falls, fractures, and motor vehicle accidents. The AGS Beers Criteria recommend avoiding all BZDs and non-BZDs, with a handful of exceptions; for example, to treat alcohol withdrawal or severe generalized anxiety. The STOPP criteria recommend limiting BZD use to less than four weeks and caution against using BZDs and non-BZDs because of increased fall risk.

- **Use of proton pump inhibitors (PPIs) for longer than eight weeks with certain exceptions for high-risk patients.** The PPI drug class includes esomeprazole (Nexium®), lansoprazole (Prevacid®), omeprazole (Prilosec®), pantoprazole

(Protonix®), and rabeprazole (Aciphex®). PPIs are among the most frequently prescribed medications in older adults. Most of these drugs are available without a prescription, which further increases their accessibility. The main concern with PPIs is that they commonly are used for longer than eight weeks in patients who do not have a high-risk situation that warrants extended use. Quite often a PPI is started during a hospital stay and then continued in error once the patient is discharged.

PPIs are perceived to be harmless and thus tend to be widely used even for minor stomach symptoms. This is true when used short-term, which is why PPIs are available OTC. Long-term use can be associated with adverse effects, though. The American Gastroenterological Association published guidelines in 2022, emphasizing the importance of using PPIs long-term only when there is a clinical diagnosis to support extended use, such as in older adults who also are taking a nonsteroidal anti-inflammatory drug (NSAID). Otherwise, use of a PPI should be limited to courses of eight weeks of therapy or less.[258] In addition, PPIs when used long-term can cause increased acid production when they are stopped abruptly. Patients misinterpret this as a return of their condition, however. Slow, gradual reduction can avoid this problem.

- **Nonsteroidal anti-inflammatory drugs (NSAIDs).** NSAIDs commonly are used to treat pain, headache, and fever. Ibuprofen (Advil®) and naproxen (Aleve®) are available without a prescription. Examples of prescription NSAIDs include diclofenac (Voltarin® and Zipsor®, among others), and meloxicam (Mobic®, among others). NSAIDs are included as PIMs because of their bleeding risk and need to be used with caution or avoided in patients with kidney impairment. They also have important interactions when combined with other medications that can cause bleeding.

As mentioned in the last point, older adults who need to use NSAIDs long-term also should be prescribed a PPI to protect against stomach bleeding.

- **Medications that are eliminated through the kidneys.** Age-related decline in kidney function, as discussed in Chapter 2, is common in older adults and an important factor that contributes to preventable adverse drug events. Medications that rely on the kidneys to be eliminated from the body need to be used in lower doses if patients have decreased kidney function. If kidney function is very poor, some medications should not be used at all.

  Examples of medications designated as PIMs based on kidney function include: NSAIDs as mentioned previously; certain antibiotics; gabapentin and pregabalin; digoxin; and anticoagulant drugs, such as apixaban, dabigatran, and rivaroxaban. It is beyond the scope of this chapter to list all of the drugs that are affected by kidney function or to provide both generic and brand names due to space. A more useful approach is for individuals who have decreased kidney function—even if due to common age-related changes—to talk with their pharmacist about their drug lists to review for appropriate dosing.

- **Use of antipsychotic medications in patients with dementia or delirium to treat behavioral symptoms of dementia** *when non-drug approaches have failed and the patient is at risk of hurting himself or others.* Aripiprazole (Abilify®), olanzapine (Zyprexa®), quetiapine (Seroquel®), and risperidone (Risperdal®) are examples of antipsychotic agents that often are prescribed to treat behaviors like agitation, restlessness, aggression, and other disruptive behaviors that can occur in later stages of dementia. Antipsychotic agents are not recommended as initial treatment because they are of limited effectiveness and associated with serious side effects. These include sedation, confusion, and an increased risk of sudden stroke and death. Antipsychotics are powerful drugs that should be turned to only after non-drug approaches and other drug therapy are unsuccessful.[259,260]

A discussion of the AGS Beers and STOPP criteria is not complete without emphasizing the following two important considerations. First, as stated earlier, the medications on the lists are *potentially* inappropriate, not *definitely* inappropriate. This means that there are situations in which a medication included on one of these PIM lists is a reasonable option for an individual. In some cases, patients might have been taking the drug without problems and are being carefully monitored for adverse effects that might develop. In other cases, there may be no other options, and a trial of the medication is warranted. The purpose of the criteria is to raise a yellow caution flag for clinicians and provide guidance before prescribing these drugs.

Second, situation and context matter. For many of the medications included in the listings, the drugs are considered inappropriate *only under certain conditions*. Each item in the listings describes when the drug or drug class is considered inappropriate and when there are exceptions to the recommendation. For example, the criteria that address proton pump inhibitors, benzodiazepines, and antipsychotics also specify exceptions for when the use of these drug classes is considered clinically appropriate. Thus, it is important to understand the context in which medications are included on the listings. Certain criteria apply only to certain patients taking those drugs.

VALUE OF POTENTIALLY INAPPROPRIATE MEDICATION LISTS

The AGS Beers Criteria and STOPP are tools for health-care professionals and have been a tremendous boon to promote safer prescribing among older adults. The AGS Beers Criteria have some advantages in the United States, and health professionals here are more likely to be familiar with this tool compared to STOPP.

The primary purpose of either list is to educate clinicians and provide clinical guideposts when prescribing for older adults. The criteria serve as a yellow caution flag as a reminder of the need for greater caution with these medications. Safer drug therapy or nondrug therapy options are encouraged when they are available.

Another value of the criteria is that they can be used by patients and health-care professionals alike as a way to open the door to a conversation about higher-risk medications. Information for consumers about the AGS Beers Criteria, along with several Tip Sheets, is available on the Health in Aging website, the consumer-facing website run by the American Geriatrics Society (https://www.healthinaging.org/medications-older-adults).

HOW OLDER ADULTS CAN USE POTENTIALLY INAPPROPRIATE MEDICATION LISTS

As an active member of your health-care team, you are your best advocate. Knowing about the PIM criteria empowers you to ask if any of your medications are considered to be potentially inappropriate based on your age. Be sure that anyone reviewing your medication list is aware of all nonprescription products you take, as some are PIMs, too. Shared decision making involves talking with your health-care providers about the expected benefits and potential harms of your medications. Can older adults safely take a medication that is "potentially inappropriate"? In many cases, yes. Should alternative medications be considered? In many cases, yes. What matters is that your drug therapy is personalized to your situation.

Ask about medication side effects and what symptoms you can watch for, especially if you take a PIM, so you can help catch a potential problem early. Be aware of new symptoms and let your physician know right away. Don't assume it is part of merely "getting older," because it could be an adverse drug reaction.

If you learn you are taking a medication that is considered potentially inappropriate, find out more about it by talking with your physician and pharmacist. Be aware that these medications can be used safely by many patients. Ask if the AGS Beers Criteria apply to your situation; some recommendations might apply only in certain circumstances. Is there a safer alternative or a nondrug option to consider? Is it possible to deprescribe (stop or reduce) a PIM you have been taking? The key is to determine with your physician and pharmacist what the optimal medication is *for you*. Never stop taking a medication without talking with either of them first, as this can be harmful. The Health in Aging website (included in the last section) has a Tip Sheet on what you can do if you are taking a PIM.[261]

Finally, you can use the three general criteria from STOPP previously described to engage with your prescribers or pharmacist about the medications you take. Namely, for each medication, confirm the reason it is prescribed; ask if the medication should be continued (and for how long); and confirm that none of your drugs are from the same drug class (to avoid duplication of a medication).

While it is safe to assume that geriatric-trained clinicians are well-versed in these tools and understand the value of applying them to the care of older adults, it is less likely that nongeriatric-trained health-care professionals will be as familiar with the AGS Beers Criteria. Thus, patients and consumers who are aware of PIMs can bring up this important topic with their prescribers. Even if you are not taking a PIM, it is valuable to have brought up the topic and to be proactive. The ultimate goal is to identify and prevent medication-related problems.

SUMMARY

Potentially inappropriate medications (PIMs) are drugs or drug classes identified by geriatrics experts for which the risks of using these drugs generally outweigh the benefits in older individuals. PIMs are recommended to be avoided when possible, as often there are safer options available. An important clarification is that PIMs are only *potentially* inappropriate, and use of these medications can be a reasonable choice for certain people.

The topic of PIMs is important because it further explains why medication use in older adults needs to be approached with greater caution. Readers are encouraged to discuss this information with their health-care professionals and should never make changes to their medications on their own. Adverse effects associated with PIMs are considered to be preventable; thus older adults and their family members should be educated on how to monitor for possible adverse effects.

The AGS Beers Criteria and the STOPP criteria are two widely accepted tools that identify PIMs and serve to educate clinicians. Patients can benefit from being familiar with these tools because they offer an opportunity to begin the conversation with their health-care team about ways to avoid high-risk medications. It is important to repeat here that a drug defined as a PIM does not mean it can never be used. Indeed, people respond differently to medications and have different health situations. Thus, a drug considered to be a PIM might be appropriate for certain patients. The next chapter continues this discussion on high-risk medications in older adults.

KEY POINTS

- Experts have defined "potentially inappropriate medications" (PIMs) as medications that have a higher risk of side effects and reduced clinical benefit in patients age sixty-five and over, and for which safer options generally are available.
- The two most respected PIM lists are the American Geriatrics Society's (AGS) Beers Criteria and STOPP (Screening Tool of Older People's Prescriptions).
- The purpose of these drug listings is to educate prescribers about the risk and benefit of medications in older adults and to be more cautious when prescribing and monitoring these medications.
- Knowing about PIMs enables patients to start conversation with their physicians and pharmacists about the risks and benefits of these medications and to ask about safer options when feasible.
- PIMs can be appropriate for use in certain situations, but patients should be educated about symptoms and side effects to watch for in order to avoid medication-related problems.

Chapter 11

High-Risk Medications in Older Adults

The potentially inappropriate medications (PIMs) discussed in the previous chapter have been identified by geriatrics experts as being high-risk in older adults in certain situations.[262] This chapter continues to explore high-risk medications by focusing on five groups of medications that have been identified through national medication use databases as having unique safety concerns in older adults.[263,264,265] As with PIMs, these medications warrant a more cautious approach, but they can be used safely and appropriately in older persons and can still be very beneficial in many situations. Knowledge of these medications provides an opportunity for older adults and family members to better appreciate the benefits and possible harms so they can work more closely with their physicians and pharmacists to ensure that these medications are used safely.

MEDICATION BENEFITS AND RISKS

One of the key principles of safe medication use is to recognize that medications have both desirable effects (benefits) and unwanted effects (risk or harms). When choosing drug therapy, physicians and patients need to consider both sides of the equation. Understanding this balance is particularly important for older individuals because they are more vulnerable to experiencing medication-related problems (as discussed in Chapter 2). For most medications, rest assured that the benefits are far greater than the potential for harm. Few drugs would be approved by the government otherwise. However, this balance can shift for selected medications in older adults, which is why we are talking about these drugs here.

The PIMs described in the previous chapter have been identified by geriatrics experts as drugs for which the risks are greater than the benefits in certain situations and for which alternative options should be used when available. This chapter introduces additional high-risk drug categories that are commonly used in older individuals. In contrast to PIMs, the benefit side of the equation can remain high for most of these medications despite important side effects, and there may not be safer alternatives available. As with PIMs, extra care is warranted when they are prescribed. Importantly, benefits and risks can look different for each person. The best drug choice will vary depending on an individual's set of circumstances. Ultimately, informed prescribers and patients need to work together to maximize the benefit side of the equation and minimize possible harms.

This information is not intended to be alarmist or to scare you away from effective drug therapy. My goal is to highlight that potential risks can be associated with commonly used medications in older adults, *and* that many of these problems can be prevented. As the concept of shared decision making takes hold, patients and family members today are expected to be more involved in health- and medication-related decisions. It is my intent that the information provided here can help with those discussions.

ANTICOAGULANT AND ANTIPLATELET DRUGS: DRUGS THAT INCREASE BLEEDING RISK

Anticoagulant drugs and antiplatelet drugs are two groups of medications that decrease the ability of the blood to clot or coagulate (thus the term "anti-coagulant"). Anticoagulants are used to treat blood clots that develop in the legs or lungs. They are highly beneficial in patients with atrial fibrillation to prevent blood clots that can cause a stroke and commonly are used in older adults for this reason. "Blood-thinners" is an informal term for anticoagulants.

Antiplatelet agents are the less-potent cousins of anticoagulants. They work by preventing platelets in the blood from sticking to each other to form a clot (thus the term "anti-platelet"). Antiplatelet drugs are used to prevent blood clots that cause strokes and heart attacks. They also are used following placement of a heart stent to prevent a clot forming around the stent. Common anticoagulant and antiplatelet drugs are listed in **Table 11-1**. Note that aspirin, which is available over-the-counter (OTC), is an antiplatelet agent.

Table 11-1. Anticoagulant and Antiplatelet Drugs

Drug name	Brand name
Anticoagulant drugs	
Warfarin	Coumadin®
Dabigatran	Pradaxa®
Apixaban	Eliquis®
Edoxaban	Savaysa®
Rivaroxaban	Xarelto®
Antiplatelet Drugs	
Aspirin*	(many)
Clopidogrel	Plavix®
Prasugrel	Effient®
Ticagrelor	Brilinta®

*Aspirin is available over-the-counter (nonprescription).

These two drug classes are considered high-risk because of the potential to increase the risk of bleeding. Data from emergency department visits in the United States have shown that serious bleeding events with anticoagulant and antiplatelet agents occur more frequently in older adults compared to younger individuals.[266] Yet these are highly beneficial drugs and widely prescribed to manage certain conditions in older adults, as mentioned above. Stroke prevention in older adults with atrial fibrillation is a great example of the value of these medications. Thus, the benefits of these drugs are high enough in most situations that they outweigh the potential harm.

To reduce the likelihood of a serious bleeding event, patient education and careful monitoring at home are key. Individuals who take a blood-thinner or antiplatelet drug need to talk with their physician and pharmacist to better understand the risk of bleeding, how to monitor for signs and symptoms, and what to do if bleeding occurs. Pharmacists can check for drug interactions and educate patients about interactions with nonprescription products. Namely, NSAIDs should be avoided, and aspirin should only be taken if instructed by a physician. Beware that aspirin can be found in OTC products as a "hidden" ingredient.

DIABETES MEDICATIONS: DRUGS THAT CAN CAUSE HYPOGLYCEMIA

Type 2 diabetes is one of the most common health conditions in older adults. It is a condition marked by impairment in how the body uses and regulates blood sugar (glucose). The result is too much sugar in the bloodstream that eventually damages blood vessels in the heart, kidneys, and eyes if not controlled. Drug therapy is one of the core pillars for managing diabetes and works by lowering blood sugar levels. There are several drug classes available that can be used to treat diabetes, some of which have the potential to cause severe hypoglycemia, or low blood sugar. Low blood sugar levels can be life-threatening. In particular, insulin and the sulfonylurea drug class have been associated with severe hypoglycemia in older adults and the need for emergency department visits.[267] These drugs fall into the high-risk category because they remain important treatment options for older adults, yet they can contribute to this important adverse event if not used properly. Insulin products and sulfonylurea drugs are listed in **Table 11-2**. As noted in the table, long-acting insulins have a much lower risk of causing hypoglycemia and are not associated with the same concerns for low blood sugars as are the fast and intermediate-acting insulins.

Table 11-2. Insulin and Oral Hypoglycemic Agents

Drug name	Brand name	Comment
Insulin products		
Lispro	Humalog®	Rapid acting
Aspart	Novolog®	Rapid acting
Glulisine	Apidra®	Rapid acting
Regular insulin	Humulin R®, Novolin R®	Short acting
NPH	Humulin N®, Novolin N®	Intermediate acting
Glargine*	Lantus®, Basaglar®, Toujeo®, others	Long acting
Detemir*	Levemir®	Long acting
Degludec*	Tresiba®	Long acting

Sulfonylurea drugs		
Chlorpropamide	Diabinese®	One of the older agents; rarely used today
Glimepiride	Amaryl®	Also a PIM
Glipizide	Glucotrol®	Also a PIM
Glyburide	Micronase®	Also a PIM

PIM = potentially inappropriate medication
*Hypoglycemia is uncommon with long-acting insulin products.

In addition, not all diabetes medications are considered to be higher-risk drugs in older adults. Many diabetes medications are associated with low or no risk of hypoglycemia. Be aware that not all injectable diabetes medications are insulin products. Thus, do not assume that if you take an injectable diabetes medicine it is insulin. If you are unsure, check with your pharmacist.

Insulin and the sulfonylurea drug class carry the potential for hypoglycemia because of the way these drugs work in the body. Without going into too much detail, these drugs increase the amount of insulin in the body, which then decreases sugar in the bloodstream. When either of these types of drugs are taken without sufficient food intake, it leads to the potential for blood sugar levels to decrease too much, causing hypoglycemia. The double whammy in older adults is that symptoms of low blood sugar can be harder to notice, which can delay identifying hypoglycemia as the problem. Initial symptoms in older individuals often are vague, such as weakness, dizziness, feeling unwell, and confusion, rather than the more traditional early symptoms such as fast heart rate and sweating.[268]

Importantly, hypoglycemia is preventable, but patients need to be properly educated about this risk and how to avoid it. Individuals need to know if they are prescribed a medication that has the potential to cause hypoglycemia and the importance of proper food intake, including the timing of eating. In addition, older adults and caregivers need to be educated about symptoms of low blood sugar to aid in early detection so as to avoid it progressing to a more serious event.

To illustrate some of these problems, one of my clients injected his third dose of fast-acting insulin (lispro) before bedtime without any food rather than with his evening meal. Fast-acting insulins are "meal-time" insulins and designed to be administered with a meal, not before bed and without food. Another client, an older adult herself, was prescribed glipizide (a sulfonylurea) daily and took it every morning; however, she was so busy caring for her mother that she neglected to feed herself regularly and often skipped breakfast. Both of these individuals experienced episodes of hypoglycemia because they did not realize the risk of low blood sugar levels and the importance of taking their medicines with food.

OPIOID PAIN MEDICATIONS

Pain is common in older adults and can affect quality of life and ability to function. Opioid pain medications can be an effective option for persons with moderate to severe pain. Often other medications are not a safe option in older persons or they are ineffective. Opioids are the most potent pain medicines available, but older adults are more likely to experience potentially serious adverse drug events with these drugs. Thus, they fall into the high-risk category because often their benefit is high; yet, the risks require careful attention. Of note, discussion about risks and benefits of opioid pain medicines does not apply when these drugs are used to treat persons with cancer or at the end of life.

The main concern in older adults is the potential for adverse effects such as constipation, nausea, sedation, falls, confusion, and delirium.[269] Opioids can cause severe constipation; thus, laxatives should be prescribed along with an opioid medicine. In addition, opioid pain medicines can have important drug interactions with benzodiazepines, gabapentin (Neurontin®), and pregabalin (Lyrica®). The combination with these medications increases the risk of severe sedation, slow and shallow breathing, and overdose.[270]

Older adults discharged from the hospital to home with an opioid prescription are at a high risk of experiencing a significant adverse event.[271] In particular, gastrointestinal issues like nausea and constipation, delirium, falls, and fractures have been reported. Many of these harms can be prevented when patients and clinicians work together to ensure that the proper dose and choice of opioid is prescribed; monitoring is in place to watch for side effects; and patients understand how to correctly take these medicines. Older adults who take opioids and their family members should be informed about interactions with other drugs and alcohol and should know about side effects and symptoms for which to watch.

ANTICHOLINERGIC DRUGS

Drugs with anticholinergic properties have been identified as PIMs and were mentioned in the previous chapter. [272,273] The potential for adverse drug events associated with this group of medications is considered to be greater than the expected benefit in older adults. Rather than referring to a drug class, the term "anticholinergic" refers to how these drugs work in the body and the side effects they produce. Drugs with anticholinergic properties are used to treat overactive bladder, COPD (chronic obstructive pulmonary disease), and Parkinson's disease. Many other drugs have anticholinergic properties as side effects and are used to treat still more conditions like depression, schizophrenia, dizziness, diarrhea, and allergies.

To better understand what this means, bear with me for a brief pharmacology lesson. Anticholinergic drugs block a specific part of our nervous system called the cholinergic system. The chemical messenger in this part of the nervous system is called acetylcholine. The cholinergic system has many effects throughout the body. It controls heart rate and how fast the gut moves, for example. It also controls memory and learning processes in the brain. Drugs that block the messenger acetylcholine have *anti*-cholinergic activity. Thus, we refer to these medications as anticholinergic drugs or drugs with anticholinergic properties.

Anticholinergic drugs are associated with anticholinergic effects that result from blocking acetylcholine throughout the body, as described.

These side effects thus include a collection of symptoms, namely dry eyes, dry mouth, constipation, urinary retention, blurred vision, sedation, decreased memory, and confusion. Older adults are more susceptible than younger persons to the effects in the brain, namely, decreased memory and confusion. This is a large part of why anticholinergic drugs are such a concern in older persons.

In particular, there is a growing amount of research that suggests a relationship between the use of anticholinergic drugs and cognitive impairment, including potentially irreversible dementia.[274] Thus, it is important to limit exposure to anticholinergic drugs as much as possible. The risk appears to be associated with taking multiple drugs with anticholinergic properties at one time, as well as cumulative use over many years. Examples of drugs that have strong anticholinergic properties are listed in **Table 11-3**.

Table 11-3. Common Drugs with Strong Anticholinergic Properties**

Generic name	Brand name	Use or drug category
Benztropine	Cogentin®	Parkinson's disease
Chlorpheniramine*	Chlor-Trimeton®, others	Antihistamine, first-generation
Cyclobenzaprine	Flexeril®	Skeletal muscle relaxant
Darifenacin	Enablex®	Overactive bladder
Diphenhydramine*	Benadryl®, others	Antihistamine, first-generation
Doxylamine*	Unisom®, others	Antihistamine, first-generation
Hydroxyzine	Vistaril®	Antihistamine

Hyoscyamine	Levsin®	Antispasmodic
Meclizine	Antivert®	Vertigo, dizziness
Olanzapine	Zyprexa®	Antipsychotic
Oxcarbazepine	Trileptal®	Antiepileptic (sometimes used to treat neuropathy)
Oxybutynin	Ditropan®	Overactive bladder
Quetiapine	Seroquel®	Antipsychotic
Solifenacin	VESIcare®	Overactive bladder
Trospium	Sanctura®	Overactive bladder

*Available over-the-counter (nonprescription)
** Please note the list is not complete.

FALL-RISK DRUGS

Fall prevention remains a topic of high interest among clinicians and public health officials alike. A fall can have devastating effects on an older adult, including the risk of hip fracture. According to the Centers for Disease Control and Prevention (CDC), falls in older adults are associated with over 34,000 deaths per year, 3 million emergency department visits, and $50 billion in medical costs.[275]

Several drug classes have been identified as fall-risk medications. These drug classes are considered to be high risk in older adults because many are appropriate choices for managing certain conditions in older adults; however, they also are associated with fall risk.[276,277] They are:

- Benzodiazepines
- Non-benzodiazepine drugs

- Antipsychotic drugs
- Certain antidepressant drug classes
- Antiepileptic drugs (seizure medications, but some also treat nerve pain or other atypical pain)
- Selected cardiovascular drugs

It is beyond the scope of this chapter to list all of the individual drug names in these drug classes. Instead, I encourage you to talk with your pharmacist or physician about your medication list to see if you are taking any of these fall-risk drugs.

Taking these medications in combination certainly is riskier than taking just one or maybe two. The AGS Beers Criteria of PIMs cautions against the use of three or more at the same time.[278] Each person will react differently. Side effects of these medications that contribute to fall risk include sedation, dizziness or feeling lightheaded when you stand up, decreased coordination or loss of balance, decreased alertness, and decreased memory. If you notice these types of symptoms, it is important to talk with your pharmacist or physician. Ask them to work with you to reduce the number of fall-risk medications or reduce the dosages. Stories about older adults who experience a drug-related fall unfortunately are too common, whether it is from a sedating muscle relaxer or because one's blood pressure was too low from taking multiple blood pressure medicines

HOW OLDER ADULTS CAN USE THIS INFORMATION ABOUT HIGH-RISK DRUG CATEGORIES

There is no magic formula that will provide a safety score for a medication. Risks and benefits of drug therapy have to be measured for each individual. The information provided here about higher-risk medications provides guideposts to encourage you to have conversations with your health-care team. Shared decision making involves talking about risks and benefits of drug therapy to make sure it is the best choice for your situation. There are many situations where these PIMs or high-risk medications will be the best choice for an individual. Rest assured, these medications can be safely used, especially when additional measures of care are taken.

Safe use hinges on careful prescribing, monitoring, and patient education. From the prescribing perspective, medications need to be dosed appropriately based on your kidney and liver function, drug interactions, and other health conditions. Without medical or pharmacy training, you are not expected to know how to properly prescribe these medications. However, you can be involved by double checking with your prescriber or pharmacist that the dose is appropriate in light of any other health conditions and that there are no important interactions.

Monitoring is a responsibility of both the clinician and patient. In between office visits, you have the important job of monitoring for side effects. This is especially important for medications discussed here that are associated with specific types of adverse events. Thus, you need to make sure you know the signs and symptoms to look for. If needed, enlist the support of a family member or friend to help keep an eye out for changes that might signal an adverse effect. If laboratory tests or other monitoring are required, stay on top of appointments to get these monitoring tests done.

Finally, patients must be educated on how to take and use their medications safely at home. Thus, take time with your pharmacist to learn about what you can do to minimize the risk of a having a serious side effect. For the high-risk medications and PIMs discussed in this and the previous chapter, awareness of possible concerns can empower you to be more engaged with your drug therapy. Ask your pharmacist about interactions with prescription and nonprescription drugs, food, or alcohol that could contribute to an adverse effect. Part V delves more deeply into these and other ways patients can be more proactive in maximizing drug benefits and reducing the risk of adverse events.

SUMMARY

Five drug categories were described that warrant extra measures of care when they are used in older individuals. These high-risk medications are uniquely challenging in older adults because they have an important role in the treatment of certain health conditions, yet they also are associated with the potential for important adverse drug events. These adverse events can be prevented when patients and family members are more engaged with their health-care team to ask questions about how to safely use and monitor these drugs. When appropriate, alternative treatments should be discussed. Knowledge about why these medications are considered to be problematic in older adults can help empower patients and family members to use them more safely. Awareness of PIMs and high-risk medications allows individuals to participate with their health-care team in choosing the safest and most effective drug therapy for their unique health situation.

KEY POINTS

- As we get older, the balance between benefit and harm for certain medications can shift, leading to an increased potential for adverse effects.
- Drugs and drug classes that are considered high-risk in older adults include anticoagulant and antiplatelet drugs, diabetes medications that cause hypoglycemia, opioid pain medicines, anticholinergic drugs, and fall-risk drugs.
- Many of the adverse drug events associated with high-risk medications can be prevented through careful prescribing, monitoring, and patient education.

Chapter 12

Prescribing Omissions: Under-Prescribing of Important Medications

Much attention has been given so far in this book to problems and concerns that arise from the use of too many medications in older individuals. This chapter shifts the focus to the opposite concern: medication underuse. Yes, despite all the conversation about medication overload and related harms, it is important to consider the possible harms that can occur when an individual is not prescribed a potentially beneficial medicine.

An estimated 40 to 67 percent of community-dwelling older adults are not receiving one or more medications that are considered to be of clinical benefit.[279,280] In addition, researchers have found that underuse of medication in older individuals is associated with negative health outcomes including cardiovascular (heart-related) events, emergency department visits, and hospitalizations.[281,282,283]

An untreated condition is one of the eight categories of medication-related problems introduced in Chapter 3. Thus, awareness of potential omissions of drug therapy is another opportunity to prevent medication-related problems. This chapter focuses on issues surrounding prescribing omissions or the under-prescribing of potentially appropriate drug therapy.

DEFINING AND IDENTIFYING POTENTIAL PRESCRIBING OMISSIONS

Potential prescribing omissions or under-prescribing is defined as the absence of a medication that is potentially beneficial in the treatment or prevention of a health condition.[284] There are several resources that clinicians can use to identify a situation where under-prescribing has occurred. One resource is the use of clinical practice guidelines. These guidelines essentially are expert recommendations of how to manage a particular health condition. However, guidelines are created for one health condition at a time. They rarely take into consideration older patients with multiple health conditions and who take multiple medications. Thus, experts agree that caution is warranted when applying clinical guidelines to an older individual. As we've already learned, if multiple guidelines are applied to one person, it can lead to excessive prescribing and complex regimens that actually could be harmful.[285]

Another resource for clinicians is a list of potential prescribing omissions developed specifically for older adults by geriatrics experts, the Screening Tool to Alert to Right Treatment, known by its acronym START. This tool is the companion document that goes with the STOPP criteria (Screening Tool of Older Persons' Prescriptions) discussed in Chapter 10.[286] The START criteria identifies medications for which benefit in older adults in certain situations is encouraged based on clinical research. Examples of the START criteria are found in **Table 12-1**. Of note, these criteria suggest medications that *potentially* should be prescribed for an individual, not that they are *definitely* needed. Every person's situation is unique, and the addition of a medication in some cases may not be the best choice for an individual. As with the use of clinical practice guidelines, clinicians need to be mindful when applying the START criteria so as to avoid medication overload.

REASONS FOR PRESCRIBING OMISSIONS

Reasons why medications are not prescribed when they theoretically could be of benefit are less well-studied. When reviewing an individual's medication list, it is easier to focus on what is on the list, rather than what is absent from it. To identify a condition that is untreated, clinicians need access to information about all of the person's health conditions. Clinicians who practice in a different health system might be excluded from such access, and most pharmacy systems are separate from medical systems; thus pharmacists typically would not have access.

Detecting a drug that is omitted requires an intentional review for this type of medication-related problem. During a brief medical visit or pharmacy encounter, omissions might be overlooked in favor of prioritizing issues related to medications the patient currently is taking. Another reason prescribing omissions occur is that physicians may already have determined that adding a certain medication is not an appropriate choice for the patient; for example, a medication might not be a good choice because of a previous adverse reaction, patient preference, or high cost. Unfortunately, some omissions occur because a prescriber thinks the patient is "too old" to benefit from treatment. This is ageism and should not be the sole reason to withhold therapy.[287]

Not all prescribing omissions need to be viewed as a problem. Clinicians and patients should always be mindful of finding the balance between taking the right combination of medications to manage a person's health conditions and taking more medications than are helpful. Recall that often there are limited numbers of older adults enrolled in clinical studies. Most medications are studied in fairly healthy participants. Thus, it is unknown how effective some drugs actually will be in an older individual who is less healthy and takes multiple medications.[288] Decisions to not prescribe potentially appropriate drug therapy need to be individualized.

VALUE OF ADDRESSING POTENTIAL PRESCRIBING OMISSIONS

Under-prescribing is raised as one of the issues that matter to older individuals because it can be associated with avoidable adverse outcomes. A study from 2017 published in the *Journal of the American Pharmacists Association* found that 13 percent of hospital admissions that were deemed preventable were related to an untreated condition that should have been identified.[289] This highlights the need to optimize drug therapy by considering both *appropriate* polypharmacy including drugs that are absent but could be beneficial as well as *inappropriate* polypharmacy and drugs that are unnecessary or harmful.

Examples of common prescribing omissions in older adults are described next and are also listed in **Table 12-1**. One of the more important and fairly common omissions is the absence of prescribing an anticoagulant drug ("blood thinner") in persons who have atrial fibrillation. Atrial fibrillation increases the risk of developing a blood clot that can cause a stroke. Anticoagulant drug therapy is beneficial in preventing a stroke in patients with atrial fibrillation, especially older individuals.

Prescribing omissions in patients with osteoporosis, a condition of weak or thin bones, are also clinically important and fairly common. Drug therapy is effective in reducing the risk of a bone fracture, including hip

Table 12-1. Examples of Potential Prescribing Omissions from the Screening Tool to Alert to Right Treatment (START)

Health Condition	Drug therapy that is of benefit in older adults
Patients who have had a stroke or heart attack	Aspirin or another antiplatelet medication
Patients with atrial fibrillation	Anticoagulant medication ("blood thinner")
Patients with heart failure	Angiotensin converting enzyme (ACE) inhibitor (such as enalapril, lisinopril, ramipril, and others)
Patients with osteoporosis	Medication to treat osteoporosis and supplementation with vitamin D and calcium

fracture, but many older adults may not receive treatment. Patients with osteoporosis also need to get enough calcium and vitamin D to ensure the prescribed medication can do its job to strengthen bones. Clarissa illustrates this problem. She was taking a once-monthly osteoporosis medication but not taking calcium or vitamin D supplements. Her dietary intake of calcium was minimal. I explained how her prescription medication needs the building blocks of calcium and vitamin D to strengthen her bones and talked with her about how much supplementation she should take. This is a unique example in that the omitted therapy involves non-prescription products. Not only do clinicians need to make sure patients are educated about the importance of these supplements, but patients need to follow through and take them every day as instructed.

Another important but commonly documented prescribing omission is the use of a statin drug, such as atorvastatin or simvastatin, in patients who have coronary artery disease (a narrowing of the blood vessels in the heart). Four years before I met with him, Willie had two stents placed in his heart to manage this health condition. His medicines included irbesartan to lower blood pressure and low-dose aspirin to prevent a heart attack or a stroke. Recommended treatment for coronary artery disease includes good control of blood pressure, aspirin to prevent a stroke or heart attack, and a statin drug to lower cholesterol. Thus, I spoke with Willie and his physician and recommended adding statin therapy for its long-term benefits.

Finally, prescribing omissions can address prevention of a health condition and not just treatment of existing conditions. Helen's situation illustrates this type of under-prescribing scenario. Helen had back pain and arthritis. She was prescribed hydrocodone with acetaminophen on a regular basis three times a day. She developed severe constipation, which is a well-known side effect of hydrocodone. The omission in Helen's case was that she was not prescribed a regular laxative to prevent constipation when hydrocodone was started. This is one of the more frequent omissions documented in studies and can be quite serious. Ideally, laxatives are started at the same time as the opioid medicine, in anticipation of this very common and important side effect.

HOW OLDER ADULTS CAN USE INFORMATION ABOUT POTENTIAL OMITTED THERAPY

Prescribing omissions are considered a preventable medication-related problem; thus it is important to be aware that under-prescribing can occur. Under-prescribing can be intentional, meaning your physician has identified a valid reason why a medication should not be prescribed for a particular situation. Or it can be unintentional and simply an oversight. Either way, it is important that you ask about potentially omitted drug therapy with every annual medication review or health check-up.

The material in this chapter ultimately needs to be shared with your health-care team who can review your medication regimen to identify potential prescribing omissions. However, it is important to prioritize medications that are of known benefit and avoid the pitfalls that can come with polypharmacy. Your medication list needs to be individualized for your situation, taking into account your health conditions and medications. If clinicians were to prescribe every potentially omitted medication, this could lead to overprescribing and related adverse outcomes. The goal therefore is to optimize your medication list so it contains the right medications for your quality of life and well-being.

To avoid a prescribing omission that could be potentially important for you, ask for a comprehensive assessment from either your primary care physician or a geriatrician (medical doctor who specializes in geriatrics). A thorough assessment can help identify health conditions for which drug therapy is not prescribed but could be of value. You also can ask for a medication review from a pharmacist with geriatrics expertise to review your medications for prescribing omissions along with other medication-related problems. Remember that pharmacists might not have access to your medical information, so have a list of your medical conditions available.

SUMMARY

Identifying prescribing omissions is a cornerstone of appropriate drug therapy and must be considered alongside the need to avoid potentially inappropriate medications and medication overload. Awareness of the important role of under-prescribing empowers individuals to be proactive and talk with their health-care team about drug therapy that may not be currently prescribed but perhaps could be of benefit. The goal ultimately is to strike a reasonable balance between taking medications that are of known clinical benefit while minimizing or avoiding those that are potentially harmful or of uncertain benefit.

KEY POINTS

- Prescribing omissions or under-prescribing refers to the absence of a medication that is potentially beneficial in the treatment or prevention of a health condition.
- Under-prescribing is associated with negative health outcomes and is considered a preventable medication-related problem.
- Identifying and addressing prescribing omissions is an essential aspect of optimizing drug therapy in older adults.
- Older adults can reduce the risk of experiencing potentially omitted drug therapy by asking their physician for a comprehensive assessment and their physician or pharmacist for a thorough medication review to identify possible under-prescribing.

Part V

Strategies for Safer Medication Use

Chapter 13

Advocate for Yourself

Suboptimal medication use is marked by overuse, underuse, and inappropriate prescribing. Older adults frequently suffer from a fragmented health-care system where care is subdivided among multiple specialists. Communication can be lacking. Absence of a universal electronic health record can hinder access to patient information between providers. Furthermore, pharmacy databases that do not communicate with those of medical or health systems place older adults at even higher risk of suboptimal medication use. The result is poorly coordinated patient care with patients caught in the middle. The Lown Institute's report *Medication Overload: America's Other Drug Problem* states, "In most cases, no single health care professional is assigned responsibility—or has the time, training, and resources—to coordinate patient care, keep track of all the drugs patients have been prescribed, and protect them from medication overload."[290] Until these health system problems are fixed, patients must take it upon themselves to advocate for ways to optimize their medication use.

Advocating requires active participation on your health-care team. As discussed earlier, you are the most important member of that team. Your input and perspective matter. Strategies to reduce excessive and unnecessary medication use among older adults call for more conversation between patients and clinicians about medications.[291] Indeed, patients can start the ball rolling by bringing up questions and talking about their drug therapy. I understand this can be intimidating for older individuals who were taught never to question their physicians. However, the way we deliver health care has shifted, and in today's complex environment, greater patient participation is expected and necessary.

This chapter is about the importance of advocating for yourself or your family member to reduce risks of medication-related problems amid a complex health system. To advocate, according to the Merriam-Webster dictionary, is to support or argue for a cause.[292] The cause in this case is your own health and well-being. If you do not voice your concerns and questions to the health-care professionals who guide your care, how will they know what matters to you? Asking about how you can avoid unnecessary and excessive medication use is one of the most valuable conversations you can have with your health-care team.

PERSON-CENTERED CARE AND SHARED DECISION MAKING

In the past two decades, health care has experienced a major shift in how care is delivered and reimbursed. This new framework is transitioning to payment based on value and quality of care rather than on a fee-for-service or quantity basis. Integral to this approach is a greater emphasis on person-centered care, which necessitates a more active role of the patient in health-care decisions. Person-centered care might be the latest buzzword in medicine, but the concept is not new. Person-centered care, also referred to as patient-centered care, represents a focus on what matters most to each individual when making health-care decisions.[293] When applied to medication use, person-centered care involves finding out what matters most to an individual regarding health care and life goals. The need to voice your preferences is discussed later in this chapter.

Shared decision making is closely intertwined with person-centered care. This concept also is not new, but has received renewed attention in recent years as the growth of value-based care has expanded beyond the hospital, to reach all settings where care is provided. Shared decision making refers to a process in which patients (and family members when needed) and clinicians together agree upon health-care decisions. It combines the health-care professional's expertise about the benefits and harms of medications (or other treatment options) with the patient's insight regarding his or her preferences and health and life goals.

Benefits of shared decision making include improved health outcomes and reduced costs because patients are more satisfied and willing to follow through with the agreed upon plan. For medication use, it is anticipated that patients will be more adherent to their drug therapy and thus achieve better health outcomes. It is important to recognize that person-centered care and shared decision making provide the perfect opening for patients to advocate for themselves regarding safer and more appropriate medication use.

BE AN ACTIVE MEMBER OF YOUR HEALTH-CARE TEAM

The concept of the health-care team with the patient at the center of the team was introduced in Chapter 1. Many patients overlook their own role as a member of this team; after all, what does the average consumer know about health care and drug therapy options? However, you are the most knowledgeable person about your body and how you feel day-to-day. As part of shared decision making, hopefully you are invested in the value of your daily drug therapy and are willing to adhere to it. Regardless of who else is involved in your care, you are the member of your health-care team who is most impacted by the medications you take regularly—both the good effects and any side effects. Thus, it is advantageous to become more actively involved with your health care and medication choices.

It is important to be realistic about the ability of our current health system to deliver care in a coordinated, team-based approach. People have expressed to me frustrations about either their own care or their parents' care, exasperated that there is no coordination between physicians and no single point-person who takes responsibility for overseeing their care. The health-care team in reality does not exist for them. While disappointing, this often is the norm. Thus, often it falls on you and family members to rally members of your team and make sure everyone is aware of your care plan, health-care goals, and preferences.

Because of the medication-related problems that can arise when multiple providers are prescribing, it is essential that you identify a member of your health-care team who will champion your medication-related needs on your behalf. It could be a pharmacist in the medical clinic or doctor's office, your community pharmacist, your primary care physician, or a specialist, for example. But it needs to be someone on your team who understands your preferences and values regarding medication use, will answer your questions, and will speak out on your behalf.

Even with moving to electronic health records in the United States, we still do not have a unified system. This hinders the ability to provide fully coordinated care. Different health systems do not interface with each other, thus limiting access to patient medical records. If any of your providers are in a different health system or have an independent practice, they might not have access to your electronic record. Thus, it is important to double check that your doctors are communicating with each other. A significant limitation in our health-care system is that community pharmacies typically do not interface with health systems; thus your pharmacist may not have access to information about changes in your medications and health conditions. You need to be the conduit of information to your pharmacy and, in some cases, between your physicians. Specific strategies are provided at the end of this chapter.

VOICE YOUR PREFERENCES

As person-centered care grows, it follows that physicians, pharmacists, and other members of the health-care team need to elicit from patients their health-related preferences and goals. Looking specifically at medications, it is helpful to know if an individual prefers to take as few drugs as possible or has no problem taking several medications. I have met patients who never question what their doctor prescribes and are open to medical interventions, including added drug therapy. Others are more minimalistic and will take a medication only when absolutely necessary. These individuals tend to prefer lifestyle changes and other non-drug ways to manage their health conditions. Still other patients are minimalists with prescription medications but take lots of dietary supplements. Each of these types of patients will have a different perspective when treatment with a new medication is recommended.

Health conditions typically have more than one option for how they can be managed. Intensive medication therapy can be an alternative to surgery for certain cardiovascular conditions, for example. For other diagnoses, lifestyle changes might be an effective option instead of starting drug therapy. Knowing your choices is essential, but so too is your ability to express what you most prefer.

COMMUNICATE WITH YOUR HEALTH-CARE TEAM

When you have a concern or question about your drug therapy, no matter how small, speak up. Communicate about what will work for you or not. This might mean reaching out to your physician or another member of your team in between scheduled office visits. An appointment every three or six months does not capture the reality of your day-to-day experiences with your medication regimen and chronic conditions. Your body can change; and a new medication or dosage might lead to a new side effect or interaction. As a member of your health-care team, you need to communicate with your team about pertinent medication-related experiences, even if that means reaching out between office visits if you notice a significant change in your health or a possible adverse reaction to a medication.

Barriers to adherence were highlighted in Chapter 8, along with the importance of discussing issues that might prevent you from taking a medication at all or from taking it according to the instructions. Cost is a common barrier, but finding ways to overcome financial barriers is possible, as long as you let your health-care team know about your concerns. If transportation is a barrier and you know you can't get to the pharmacy for a week to pick up an important new medication, let someone help you figure out a solution. If you are instructed to make an important lifestyle change, such as starting an exercise program or quitting smoking, be honest about what you can or cannot take on. Some people can get motivated after a health scare, while others feel too overwhelmed. If you don't think you can follow through on a recommended treatment (drug therapy or nondrug), it is best to be truthful.

The goal is to have an honest conversation with your physician about drug therapy options and what you are willing to do to manage your health. It does not help anyone if you say "yes" to your health-care team but "no" inside your head. Not adhering to your drug therapy plan leads to wasted time and money, as discussed in Chapter 8. Find a way to not feel intimidated in communicating with your healthcare team. Ask questions, share relevant day-to-day experiences that trouble you about a medication, and double check that your health-care providers are all on the same page with the medications you are taking. As you become a more active member of your health-care team, it will become easier to express your preferences and participate in person-centered care.

BE INFORMED

Shared decision-making requires that you learn about your treatment options and share in the process of deciding on a care plan. Having basic information about your health conditions and medications is essential. Your health-care professionals are the medical experts on your team and likely your primary source of information. Depending on the nature of the options and your health situation, it might be helpful to get a second opinion. Remember that your pharmacist is an excellent resource for objective drug information. If you seek information from internet sources, be careful to use only the most trustworthy websites and double check the information with a health professional you trust. There is room for caution on the internet due to unreliable websites. Recommendations on how to evaluate the quality of information from the internet is discussed in Chapter 19.

Below are four questions that offer a foundation to help you understand your treatment choices:

1. What is my diagnosis?
2. What are the treatment options? (Options might include drug therapy, nondrug therapy, and surgical or other "invasive" procedures.)

3. What are the expected benefits and potential harms of these options?
4. What happens if I do not treat the condition?

For some health conditions, there may be several options; for others only one or two. In some situations, a watch and wait approach might be reasonable. Thus, asking what might happen if you choose not to treat can shed light on the severity of the diagnosis and the value of treatment.

To illustrate how these questions might apply to drug therapy, consider the example of a patient who experiences chest pain after doing yard work and is diagnosed with a heart condition. The answers might go something like this:

1. The diagnosis is coronary artery disease caused by decreased oxygen flow to the heart muscle.
2. The drug therapy options to manage it include aspirin, a beta-blocker such as metoprolol, and a statin such as atorvastatin.
3. The benefits are that the drug therapy will prevent chest pain and a potential future heart attack. Harms include possible side effects, but not all patients will experience side effects. Aspirin can increase the risk of bleeding; some patients experience dizziness or tiredness with metoprolol and it can slow the heart rate; side effects of atorvastatin are uncommon but can include diarrhea or stomach upset, and rarely muscle pain.
4. Not treating coronary artery disease means that you will continue to have episodes of chest pain that can worsen and eventually lead to a heart attack.

These answers focus on drug therapy options for brevity and are not comprehensive. However, you can see how this information gives the patient a better understanding of the role and value of drug therapy. Additional discussion needs to include other medical or surgical treatment options, nondrug treatment options, and the patient's preferences and health-care goals.

FIND A GERIATRICIAN WHEN NEEDED

As you age and perhaps develop new health conditions that require more medications, it is important to have a physician you trust. Your physician should be attuned to the many aspects that impact healthy aging—physical, social, and emotional. Caring for patients who have multiple medical conditions, polypharmacy, and age-related physiological changes requires special skills. Not all primary care physicians have the experience and expertise to care for aging patients, and unfortunately, ageism can be present among health-care professionals.

Recall from Chapter 1 that geriatricians are physicians who specialize in working with patients who are age sixty-five and over. They can be primary care providers or serve as consultants. Not every older adult needs the expertise of a geriatric specialist. However, the input of a geriatrician can be invaluable when multiple health issues appear, symptoms begin to overlap, and treatment of one condition affects the symptoms of another condition. A "less is more" philosophy often is warranted in older adults but is not mainstream in medical training.

An important aspect of managing health conditions as we age is to find the balance between optimizing treatment so patients can remain as independent as possible while avoiding drug regimens that are overly burdensome or that cause adverse effects. Having a physician who is aware of and responsive to your overall well-being can help reach the right balance in your medical care. Thus, advocating for safe medication use might mean finding a geriatrician to join your health-care team.

SUMMARY

In this chapter, I described several ways to advocate for the safe use of your medications. Actively participating in your health care means that you need to speak up for your preferences, voice your concerns, and, when appropriate, respectfully question treatment options. It is essential that you view yourself as an integral participant on your health-care team. The following checklists will guide you on ways to advocate for yourself to more safely use medications.

What You Can Do at Home

- Choose to become more engaged in your health care and medical decisions.
- Make a list of your questions to bring to each doctor visit.
- Write down observations, symptoms, and concerns in between office visits; don't rely on your memory.
- Make notes about nondrug treatments or activities that work for you to improve or manage symptoms and also those that do not seem to help.
- Keep a diary of the progress or improvement of your medical condition and whether you think the drugs are helping (or not).
- Keep a current medication list that you carry with you at all times (see Chapter 15, **Box 15-1**); be sure it includes prescription drugs, over-the-counter products, and supplements.

What You Can Do with Your Pharmacist

- Make sure your pharmacist always has access to your complete medication list.
- Request a medication review to identify medication-related problems, including potentially inappropriate medications for older adults and undertreated conditions.
- Find out more about how the effectiveness of the medicine compares to possible side effects; that is, explore the benefits and harms for your medication.
- Ask about nondrug options that can help your medicines be more effective and/or reduce the need for drug therapy.
- Speak up about any questions or concerns regarding your drug therapy; be sure you understand enough about your medications to take them correctly.

What You Can Do with Your Physician

- Ask questions about your health conditions and treatment options, including nondrug options.
- Share your complete medication list with each physician.
- Voice your preferences about your approach to your health care.
- Review medications along with your health conditions to identify unnecessary drug therapy and possible untreated conditions.
- Bring notes with you about any changes and observations since your last appointment.
- Bring paper and pen (or a family member) so you can take notes at your appointment; ask your doctor to spell out new terminology or write it down for you.
- Confirm that your doctors are communicating with each other about your health care.
- Ask where you can learn more about your health condition or the treatment options.
- Ask for a second opinion or find a geriatrician when needed.

RESOURCES

- Agency for Healthcare Research and Quality—Videos and downloadable material to encourage patient engagement:
  - https://www.ahrq.gov/patients-consumers/index.html.
  - https://www.ahrq.gov/patients-consumers/patient -involvement/index.html
- BeMedWise—Various resources about safe medication use: http://www.bemedwise.org/
- Choosing Wisely—Lists of medical tests, treatments, and procedures that should be questioned by patients and

physicians; goal is to promote conversations and patient engagement: www.choosingwisely.org

- Choosing Wisely statements by pharmacy organizations
  - o American Society of Consultant Pharmacists (specific to older adults): https://www.choosingwisely.org/societies /american-society-of-consultant-pharmacists/
  - o American Society of Health-system Pharmacists: https://www.choosingwisely.org/societies /american-society-of-health-system-pharmacists/
- World Health Organization, Medication without Harm patient engagement tool
  - o 5 Moments for Medical Safety (downloadable brochure of questions to ask): https://www.who.int/initiatives /medication-without-harm

Chapter 14

Know Your Medications

When I ask my clients what medications they take, it is not uncommon to hear responses along the lines of, "I take the blue pill at 8 a.m. and the yellow one at bedtime." Others might know the names of most of their medications but not know why they are taking them. "It's what my doctor prescribed," is a common answer. One of the fundamental tenets of safe medication use is to know basic facts about the medications you take. There are eight essential items I focus on, as summarized in **Box 14-1**.

Having a basic understanding of the drugs you take every day can go a long way to improve adherence and help you avoid duplicated therapy,

---

Box 14-1. Eight Essential Items of Medication Information

1. The brand and generic names of the medication
2. Reason for taking the medication
3. Instructions for how and when to take the medication
4. How to handle a missed dose
5. How long to take the medication and if refills are needed
6. Common side effects and serious side effects
7. Important interactions, including other medicines, food, and alcohol
8. How to store the medication

unnecessary medications, and serious adverse drug events. So many of the preventable medication-related problems and medication errors that have been discussed in earlier chapters can be traced back to a lack of knowledge about one's medications. Hopefully that alone will encourage you to learn a little more about the medications you take. Next, each of these eight items are described to provide a sense of why each one matters.

BRAND AND GENERIC NAMES

Every medication has a generic name and a brand name. Individuals ideally should be familiar with both, as it can avoid confusion that can contribute to an error. There always is just one generic name; however, there can be more than one brand name, also referred to as a trade name. Generic names typically are long, multisyllabic, and a mouthful to pronounce. Few will disagree that it is easier to say Lasix® than furosemide. Combination products can be even more challenging to pronounce and remember: Symbicort® is far less confusing than formoterol/budesonide. The generic name of a drug remains constant, while different manufacturers will have different branded names. For example, generic lisinopril has the brand names of Prinivil® and Zestril®. Likewise, generic diltiazem can be sold as Cardizem®, Cartia XT®, or Tiazac®. As a result, the common medication "language" used in pharmacies and by pharmacists generally is that of generic names. They provide clarity, consistency, and avoid commercial bias.

Brand names are the proprietary or trademarked names given to a medication by the pharmaceutical manufacturer. All drugs when first approved by the FDA have a defined time period during which only the brand name product can be sold, with no generic options available. Thus, newly approved drugs have no competition and are more expensive. Once the period of exclusive marketing ends and the patent expires (these can be on different timelines), other manufacturers can make and sell a generic version of that same medication.[294] A generic medication offers a less expensive but equally safe and effective option to a brand name product. Unfortunately, drug pricing in recent years has become extremely controversial, with the cost of several generic products experiencing significant unexplained increases. Discussion of drug pricing is beyond the scope of this book, but the topic will continue to garner attention in the coming years.

Knowledge of both the generic and brand names of your medications can help avoid medication errors at home. Drug lists provided by different medical offices, clinics, pharmacies, hospitals, or rehabilitation facilities might use the generic or brand names interchangeably. When a patient reads "amlodipine" on one list and "Norvasc" on another, an unknowing patient or caregiver will not recognize these are the same drug. I recall a patient years ago who was taking one tablet of levothyroxine every morning along with one tablet of Synthroid. She had come home from the hospital with a bottle of levothyroxine and continued to take her Synthroid® that she had at home from before the hospitalization. These are the same drug, however: levothyroxine is the generic name of Synthroid. The patient did not know this and accidentally was taking a double dose of her thyroid medicine.

REASON FOR THE MEDICATION

Knowing why a medication is prescribed is another key fact to know about your drug therapy. You might recall that one of the criteria included in the STOPP list of potentially inappropriate medications (PIMs) from Chapter 10 is that every medication should have a valid clinical reason for use.[295] Another term that refers to the reason a drug is prescribed is "indication." So, in other words, every medication you take should have a valid indication that justifies why you are taking it; for example, a valid clinical indication for valsartan is to treat high blood pressure or heart failure.

Some drugs can be used to treat more than one condition. Digoxin can be used to manage heart failure or a heart rhythm disturbance. Several antiepileptic drugs can be used to treat seizures as well as nerve pain. Montelukast is approved to treat both allergies and asthma, and it should be taken either in the morning or in the evening, depending on the indication. Thus, it can be helpful to know why each drug is prescribed, especially if you need to discuss your medications with a health professional that may not have access to your medical record.

There are myriad examples that illustrate the importance of knowing the reason for each medication (along with the drug name). I had a patient who did not start a new medication for his Parkinson's disease symptoms because he did not realize what it was for. Another patient was told by his physician to stop taking his cholesterol medicine, but he continued taking simvastatin because he did not know which drug the doctor was talking about. A large portion of my patients continue diligently to take their medications without knowing why some or all of them are prescribed. "That's what the doctor gave me to take," I often hear.

There is broad value in knowing the reason for your medications. It can help motivate you to take them regularly (improve adherence) and thus improve health outcomes. It can help you better understand what to watch for at home to help your health-care team assess if the medications are helpful. In turn, this can reduce the risk of continuing drug therapy that is ineffective. Knowing the reason also can help avoid duplicated medications, either with two prescription drugs or with prescription and over-the-counter (OTC) drugs. One of my clients had prescription bottles for both omeprazole and pantoprazole, medications from the same drug class that worked in the same exact way—proton pump inhibitors (PPIs) for reducing stomach acid—but from two prescribers who were unaware of what the other prescribed. If my client had known the reason for these medications, this duplication could have been caught earlier. Still one more value of knowing the reason for your medications is to serve as a final check when you pick up a new prescription. It empowers you as the patient to confirm with the pharmacist that you are receiving the correct medication for the correct indication.

INSTRUCTIONS FOR HOW TO TAKE THE MEDICATION

Knowing the instructions for how to correctly take a medication often means more than simply being able to read the label on the prescription bottle. Instructions that seem straightforward to a health-care professional can be vague for a layperson to interpret. Does "take three times a day" mean every eight hours, or with breakfast, lunch, and bedtime? Does "take with food" mean just before eating or waiting until the meal is finished? How do you define "empty stomach"? Taking two tablets at one time is not the same as taking one tablet two times daily. Etc., etc., etc. It is frustrating to learn after the fact that you have been taking a medication incorrectly that caused it to not work or reduce its effectiveness. Certain medications have very specific instructions on when and how they need to be taken that can affect clinical outcome. Levothyroxine absorption can be significantly decreased if taken at the same time as a calcium supplement; certain oral medications for treating osteoporosis must be taken on an empty stomach and only with water or they will not be absorbed. These above examples hopefully illustrate how medication instructions sometimes can be ambiguous and the importance of making sure you are clear on what they mean.

Thus, as an extra measure of caution, read the instructions on the prescription bottle when you pick it up for the first time, with each refill, and at home before you take it (or fill a pill organizer with it). Ask the pharmacist to clarify if anything is unclear. Even when picking up a refill of a prescription, it doesn't hurt to be careful. Errors can occur if the pharmacy computer system has older and current prescriptions in your profile for the same medication. I saw a situation once where the physician had sent in a new prescription with updated instructions for furosemide two times daily, but an older version with once-daily instructions had not been inactivated and was refilled by accident. Once you walk out of the pharmacy with a prescription, it is standard practice that it cannot be returned.

WHAT TO DO IF YOU MISS A DOSE

How to handle a missed dose is another important fact to know. Hopefully, it does not happen too often, but invariably it will for most individuals. What to do if you forget to take a dose of a medication will depend on the particular drug and how many times a day it should be taken. There are two general rules of thumb regarding missed doses that will apply to *most* situations—however, there are exceptions to these rules! Always check the specific instructions you have been given for your medication.

The first general rule is that if you remember your missed dose within two hours of the scheduled time, it is okay to take it right away when you remember. The second general rule is to never double up on a drug and take two doses together. The best guidance, of course, is to check with your pharmacist when in doubt.

HOW LONG TO TAKE THE MEDICATION

It is important to know the intended duration of use for your medications. Only a small number of diagnoses are treated, cured, and no longer need drug therapy. Infections are the most common example of a condition that we actually can cure and treat with a limited duration of therapy. Most other health conditions are managed over the long-term, and drug therapy must be continued for months or years. Chronic health conditions like heart failure, coronary artery disease, or chronic obstructive pulmonary disease (COPD) require lifelong drug therapy. Other conditions might need treatment for several months, such as when treating anemia or a stomach ulcer.

Taking a medication for longer than is clinically necessary (when the duration of use is well-defined) is a signal of potentially inappropriate medication use, as mentioned in Chapter 10 from the STOPP criteria.[296] Nonsteroidal anti-inflammatory drugs (NSAIDs) and PPIs are examples of drugs that in most situations are recommended to be used only for a limited duration. In contrast, drugs for managing chronic conditions need to be refilled regularly and typically continued long-term. One of my patients started a new cholesterol medication for one month but did not continue it after the bottle was empty. When I asked her about it, she said no one told her that she needed to continue taking it.

Physicians will indicate on each prescription whether refills are needed and how many are allowed. The refill information is always found on the prescription bottle on the pharmacy's label. It's always a good idea to confirm with your physician and pharmacist how long you need to take the drug and if you need to get it refilled.

IMPORTANT SIDE EFFECTS

Essentially every medication has side effects. As a patient, it is important to know which side effects are minor and fairly common so you will not be alarmed if you notice symptoms. Knowledge is power, and this knowledge can prepare you to handle a minor side effect, should it occur. These can be bothersome but are not life-threatening. Examples include nausea, diarrhea, and constipation; drowsiness or sedation; and insomnia. Adjusting the timing of the medication often can reduce or "manage" the side effect. For example, to avoid stomach-related side effects (nausea, stomach pain), confirm with your pharmacist if it is okay to take the medication with food. If a drug causes drowsiness or sedation, perhaps it can be taken at bedtime, or if it causes insomnia, it could be taken in the morning. Of note, some side effects might seem minor but can lead to significant consequences in older individuals; thus it is important to talk about side effects with your clinicians. A good example is dry mouth, which can lead to tooth decay and gum disease, mouth sores, and difficulty eating that can ultimately affect nutritional intake.[297]

However, it also is important to be educated about less common but more severe side effects (adverse drug effects) so you can identify early any serious issues and contact your physician or pharmacist immediately. Examples of serious side effects include severe allergic reactions, bleeding, hypoglycemia, jaundice, or sudden decrease in the amount of urine produced.

It is important for you—and family caregivers who are assisting with your medications—to be educated about both common side effects and serious ones. For serious side effects, you should know what symptoms to watch for that would indicate an important side effect and what you or your caregiver should do if a symptom occurs. Drugs can cause allergic reactions, as well. Allergic reactions can range from itching and rash to anaphylactic reactions that involve swelling of the throat and difficulty breathing. Anaphylactic reactions are life-threatening and require immediate medical attention.

IMPORTANT INTERACTIONS

Drug interactions are a significant source of preventable medication-related problems. With any new prescription, the physician and pharmacist should review for interactions with your current medication list and health conditions. This is a key role for pharmacists. But pharmacists need to know about any nonprescription drugs you take, so these can be screened for interactions, too. Individuals have the responsibility to prevent drug interactions at home. Namely, be aware of possible interactions between your medications and food, alcohol, or nonprescription products (OTC products and dietary supplements), and even cannabis. Drug interactions were discussed in more detail in Chapter 9.

HOW TO STORE THE MEDICATION AT HOME

Finally, the eighth essential item to know about your medications is proper storage. Especially with injectable medications, it is important to know how to store them at home, if they need refrigeration, and how long refrigerated medications can be left at room temperature. The general recommendation for oral medications (medications taken by mouth) is to store them in a cool, dry place, away from heat and humidity. The traditional "medicine cabinet" in the bathroom is not a good spot due to the humidity from showering; nor is a cabinet above the stove where heat and steam can reach.

Although less common, certain medications must be kept in their original containers from the manufacturer and not placed into a pill organizer. Dabigatran, a drug that prevents the blood from clotting (it is one of the "blood thinners") falls into this category and cannot be added to a pill organizer because of extreme sensitivity to moisture.[298] Years ago, I consulted with a daughter who was managing her mom's medications. She used a weekly organizer for all of her mom's medications, including dabigatran, unaware of this requirement. Fortunately, her mom did not experience a serious problem. The daughter corrected the error, thus ensuring her mom was getting the full benefit of the medication going forward. Thus, storage of a medication might seem like a minor issue; however, it can impact the effectiveness of medications and is important to know.

SUMMARY

This chapter presented eight items of essential information that everyone should know about the medications they take. Having a solid understanding of one's medications can help reduce the risk of errors and medication-related problems. The material in this chapter provides a guide for what information is important and why, and it can empower patients to learn more about their medications. In turn, individuals will be better able to manage their medications safely and take them on a regular basis.

What You Can Do at Home

- Make a list of your medications that includes brand and generic names and the reason for each medication that you take.
- Keep your medication list easy to access, especially for emergency situations; for example, post in on your refrigerator.
- Read the medication label each time before taking the medicine (and when placing it in a pill organizer); make sure you have the right drug at the right time.
- Keep the pharmacy's phone number on hand so you can call with questions about side effects or what to do if you miss a dose, for example.

What You Can Do with Your Pharmacist

- Say "yes" when you are asked at the pharmacy pick-up counter if you want to speak with the pharmacist about your medication.
- Have the pharmacist explain the eight essential items to know for each of your medications (see **Box 14-1**).
- Ask for information in writing so you can review it later.

What You Can Do with Your Physician

- Make sure you know the name of each medication and why it is prescribed for you.
- Ask about common side effects as well as serious side effects; know what symptoms to look for and what you should do if they occur.
- Make sure you are clear about instructions for how and when to take the medication; write them down before leaving the office visit.
- When a new medication is prescribed, ask your physician about refills and how long you need to take it; confirm when you need to make a follow-up appointment to assess safety and/or effectiveness of the medicine.

RESOURCES

- National Institute on Aging, Safe Use of Medications in Older Adults: https://www.nia.nih.gov/health /safe-use-medicines-older-adults

- World Health Organization, Medication without Harm patient engagement tool
  - ○ 5 Moments for Medical Safety (downloadable brochure of questions to ask): https://www.who.int/publications/i/item/WHO-HIS-SDS-2019.4 or https://www.who.int/initiatives/medication-without-harm

Chapter 15

Prevent Medication Errors

Reducing medication errors is a key component of patient safety initiatives across health-care systems nationwide and globally. Although rare, some medication errors can be extremely serious. Fortunately, the vast majority of errors have minimal or no clinical consequences. By definition, all medication errors are preventable. Thus, it is important for patients and family members to understand the nature and scope of this key aspect of medication safety so they can be part of ongoing efforts to reduce the risk of serious errors and potentially harmful events.

While medication errors can occur in patients of any age, older adults have a higher risk of experiencing a medication error, in large part because they typically are exposed to more medications. Other contributing factors include the presence of multiple health conditions and age-related changes in how the body handles and responds to medications (referring to the pharmacokinetic and pharmacodynamic changes described in Chapter 2).[299] In addition, any time a person transitions from one setting of care to another, such as when a person moves between home and the hospital or between different medical specialists, there is an increased risk of triggering a medication error.

In 1999, a report by the Institute of Medicine (IOM), "To Err is Human: Building a Safer Health System," sparked a national interest in health safety and medication errors.[300] The report was a wake-up call for health systems nationwide to improve safety processes in the delivery of health care. Reducing medication errors is an essential component of this national focus, with initial efforts geared toward the hospital and nursing home settings. More recently, efforts to reduce medication errors have expanded into the community setting, where the vast majority of patients—including older adults—reside.[301,302] However, further reduction in errors in this setting can only be achieved when patients and family caregivers take a more proactive role regarding their medication use.[303,304]

DEFINING MEDICATION ERRORS

In its simplest definition, a medication error is a mistake related to drug therapy that occurs at any point during the medication use process, which is discussed in more detail below. Medication errors by nature stem from human actions or lack of actions at some point when medications are prescribed, dispensed, taken, or monitored. It is relevant to note that patients, along with physicians and pharmacists, are involved at different stages in the medication use process and thus can contribute to medication errors. As already mentioned, all errors are considered to be preventable. Many of the medication-related problems described in Chapter 3 can be considered medication errors when they involve *preventable* events.

Importantly, medication errors are not all harmful; 99 percent are minor and do not impact patient care or health outcomes. Most are never even noticed by the patient or health-care team.[305] A good chunk of errors are caught and corrected before ever reaching the patient, and thus lead to no harm. Finally, only about 1 percent of medication errors actually reach the patient and cause harm.[306] These errors are the major focus of medication safety initiatives. Prevention efforts require an all-hands-on-deck approach, including patients being engaged on their health-care team.[307]

PREVALENCE OF MEDICATION ERRORS

Differences in how medication errors are defined, tracked, and measured make it hard to gauge how often medication errors occur. By one estimate, 1.5 million medication errors occur overall in the United States every year.[308] Other estimates that focus just on individuals age sixty-five and older suggest that roughly 530,000 medication errors occur annually[309] and are associated with $887 million in health-care expenditures.[310] Based on data collected through poison control centers, the rate of medication errors per 100,000 persons in the community setting is reported to have doubled between 2000 and 2012.[311] The most common errors involved incorrect doses (a type of prescribing error), taking the wrong drug, and taking a medication twice (types of adherence errors).[312] The documented increase in medication errors is of great concern because of the sheer numbers of individuals who reside in the community setting, many of whom are older adults.

Of note, patients and consumers are encouraged to report medication errors. Two ways to access medication error reporting programs are provided in the Resources section of this chapter. Reporting errors, even if no harm occurred, is of value because it can help identify trends or sources of errors that can be corrected to prevent harmful errors in the future.

WHERE MEDICATION ERRORS OCCUR

Medication errors can occur at any point during the medication-use process. In the community setting, this process is defined by four stages: prescribing, dispensing, administration (adherence), and monitoring. These stages are depicted in **Figure 15-1**, along with the major safety checks for each. Safeguards throughout the medication-use process continually are being added and refined in efforts to improve patient safety and reduce errors. Several of these safeguards include electronic prescribing, advanced software programs that screen for interactions or dosing errors, automated alerts for prescribers, special labeling to avoid sound-alike and look-alike errors, and use of bar code scanning.

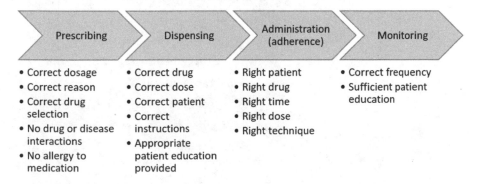

Figure 15-1. The Medication Use Process and Safety Checks for Each Stage

Examples of medication errors that coincide with each stage of the medication-use process are provided in **Table 15-1** with additional information below. Medication errors among older adults in the community setting occur most frequently in the prescribing and monitoring stages, followed by adherence-related errors. Dispensing-related errors occur least often and make up less than 2 percent of errors.[313]

Table 15-1. Examples of Medication Errors

Stage of medication-use process	Examples of medication errors
Prescribing	• Drug for which the patient has a known allergy • Drug that is ineffective for the condition • Drug that is high-risk (risks generally outweigh benefits) or high-alert • Drug with significant drug or disease interaction • Dosage that is dosed too high or too low • Unnecessary drug
Dispensing	• Dispensing an incorrect drug • Providing incorrect instructions • Refilling a prescription that has been discontinued • Filling a prescription for the wrong patient • Giving a correctly filled prescription to the wrong person at the point of sale • Providing instructions to cut the tablet in half, but the tablet is not scored (therefore not intended to be split)

Administration and adherence	• Taking the wrong drug or wrong dose
	• Taking someone else's medicine
	• Taking a medicine twice
	• Forgetting to take a medicine
	• Confusing sound-alike or look-alike names (for example metformin and metoprolol or hydralazine and hydroxyzine)
	• Forgetting to pick up a refill or not filling a new prescription
	• Stopping the medicine too early
	• Wrong timing (for example, morning instead of bedtime; taking it with or without food)
	• Continuing to take a medication despite side effects
	• Using improper technique for an inhaler or eye drops leading to insufficient drug being administered
Monitoring	• Inadequate monitoring of drug therapy or patient response (for example, clinician not checking electrolytes, drug levels, or kidney or liver function)
	• Not taking action on laboratory results (patient or clinician)
	• Not adhering to monitoring instructions at home (for example, checking blood glucose before mealtime insulin, checking daily weight with heart failure)
	• Not following up with recommended monitoring (for example, patient is asked to get a blood test or an eye exam)

Medications that more commonly have been associated with prescribing errors in older adults include certain cardiovascular medications, diuretics (water pills), insulin, oral diabetes medicines that can cause hypoglycemia, anticoagulants, acetaminophen, and nonsteroidal-anti-inflammatory drugs (NSAIDs).[314,315,316] Notably, most of these drugs were highlighted previously as high-risk or problematic drugs in older adults, thus reiterating the need for caution when prescribing and taking these medications. Wrong dose or wrong drug selection errors can result, for example, when prescribers do not have full access to a patient's medication list and medical information. Acetaminophen and NSAIDs are available without a prescription; thus they have the added potential for errors if prescribers are not aware that patients are taking these medications, for example.

To protect against dispensing errors, there are multiple safeguards in place that help pharmacists and pharmacy technicians reduce medication errors. Steps that patients can take are included later in the chapter. Pharmacists regularly receive warnings about and remain vigilant to sound-alike, look-alike medications, especially when new drugs are approved. Examples abound: Navane and Norvasc, glyburide and glipizide, bupropion and buspirone, alprazolam and lorazepam. To avoid wrong-patient errors—giving a correctly filled prescription to the wrong patient at the point of sale—it is recommended to ask for two identifiers when picking up a prescription, such as birthdate, phone number, or address.

Errors related to adherence are a major concern in the community setting, where patients are responsible for managing their own medications (or with the assistance of a caregiver). For simplicity, they are grouped with administration-stage errors. Many of the examples of nonadherence discussed in Chapter 8 also are medication errors; thus you will note similarities in the examples listed in **Table 15-1**. Common adherence errors include taking the wrong dose or wrong drug or taking a medication twice. Thus, efforts to improve adherence go hand-in-hand with reducing medication errors.

The monitoring stage of drug therapy is necessary to evaluate both safety and effectiveness. Both physicians and patients share this responsibility. Many of the reported monitoring-related errors involve clinicians not ordering needed monitoring tests (such as blood tests) or not following up with the test results. However, patients can reduce monitoring errors by being informed about what kind of monitoring is needed and following up with their physicians on results (for example, confirm if a blood test showed any abnormal values). Certain health conditions require at-home monitoring, such as checking blood sugar levels or weighing yourself daily. These at-home monitoring guidelines are a way to reduce errors, as well.

Eleanor was a seventy-seven-year-old client whose story is rather unusual, but it illustrates a range of medication errors. Eleanor was doing fairly well living alone and managing several health conditions. She took twelve medications, including the antibiotic cephalexin. She had been taking it every day, four times a day for the past two months. Usually, a course of antibiotics is limited to one to two weeks unless something more severe is going on. Her dose was within the "normal" range, but too high for this individual with reduced kidney function. She did not know that it was an antibiotic and had no idea why it might have been prescribed for her. The pharmacy had a valid prescription for cephalexin from Eleanor's physician and filled it correctly, but had no further information about why there were refills on it. The story became more peculiar when her physician did not have record of the prescription in Eleanor's profile. Clearly this was a medication error, but I could only speculate where the system breakdown occurred that led to the error. Eleanor was lucky because the error did not appear to cause an adverse drug reaction and was resolved.

IMPORTANCE OF TRANSITIONS OF CARE

Transitions of care are a particularly high-risk time for medication errors and thus deserve special attention. Transitions of care refer to any time a patient moves between different settings; for example, moving from home to a hospital, or moving from the hospital to a rehabilitation facility. Transitions also occur when patients move between primary care and specialty physicians or other providers. Common causes of medication errors associated with transitions include rushed communication, incomplete medication lists, and discrepancies between medication lists on record at one location of care and the actual list that reflects what the individual is taking at home. Similarly, discrepancies can occur between medication lists that two doctor's offices have on record for a patient. Common examples of transition of care-related medication errors include medications that are omitted from the patient's list that should be included; medications that should have been stopped but still appear on the list; and incorrect dosages.

Accurate medication lists are key to preventing medication errors. Clinicians use a process called medication reconciliation to confirm a patient's most current medication list. When discharged home from the hospital, for example, the process involves comparing the patient's discharge medication list with what the patient was taking before being hospitalized to detect and correct discrepancies and avoid errors. Medication reconciliation can and should occur at each doctor visit, as well. Thus, always keep with you a current medication list that reflects what you are taking at home.

The remainder of this chapter addresses strategies to prevent medication errors. If these strategies sound familiar, they are. Preventing medication errors is closely intertwined with reducing the risk of medication-related problems described elsewhere.

BE ENGAGED AND ASK QUESTIONS

Being engaged involves asking questions and communicating with your health-care team. Patient engagement is now a recognized key pillar to improve medication safety. Family members or friends who support you with your medications also need to be involved. The World Health Organization states in its *Medication Errors* report, "Empowering and encouraging patients to speak up, for example when something does not seem right or when a symptom is inadequately explained, can be fundamental to improving patient safety. Family members play a key role as advocates and informal carers and therefore supporting and educating them can help to improve safety."[317] Your safety matters. Even though you might feel uncomfortable at first, it is important to speak up.

Multiple prescribers and poor communication between physicians are risk factors for experiencing an error. Several of my clients have mentioned that their specialists only ask about the medications they have prescribed. Therefore, confirm that your prescribers are communicating with each other regarding your treatment plan and any changes. They will appreciate your concern.

Share your complete medication list with every prescriber, especially before a new medication is added. To avoid the prescribing cascade, ask your prescriber if the new medication might actually be treating an adverse reaction to an existing medication. If the new medication is identified as potentially inappropriate or high risk in older adults, ask if there are other options. If not, know that these medications can be used safely with a little more attention to watching for side effects and avoiding important interactions (see Chapters 9 and 10). Thus, always find out what signs or symptoms you can look for at home to make sure your medications are safe and effective. Finally, confirm with your physician or pharmacist that you are on an appropriate dose for your age and kidney function.

TALK WITH YOUR PHARMACIST

Whenever I am in line as a customer at a pharmacy, I take note of how people respond when the pharmacy technician asks customers picking up a prescription if they have any questions for the pharmacist. I have yet to hear anyone answer yes; however, this is one of the most important times to say "yes." Talking with your pharmacist when you pick up a medication is the best way to defend against errors. As stated on the Institute for Safe Medication Practices website: "Patients can play a vital role in preventing medication errors when they have been encouraged to ask questions and seek answers about their medications before drugs are dispensed at a pharmacy or administered in a hospital."[318] Having sufficient knowledge about your medications helps prevent errors at home.

Say "yes" at the pharmacy counter when you pick up a new prescription or even a refill. Even a brief exchange of information about your prescription might allow the pharmacist to uncover something amiss. If you are experiencing side effects that do not match up with the medication you are prescribed, it could signal a wrong-drug error, for example. I continually am reminded of the value of these conversations when I discover an error or problem that had gone undetected for a client. Too often, these opportunities are missed due to our disjointed and often hurried healthcare process. Take the example of a gentleman who stopped taking his heart medicine diltiazem because he thought it was the cause of his diarrhea. The actual cause of diarrhea was the diabetes medicine metformin, but his error of stopping an important heart medicine was only uncovered when I talked with him about his medications and explored what he understood about each one.

For a new medication, make sure you know the essential information, as described in Chapter 14. This is your chance to compare the information you got from your physician at the office visit with what your pharmacist explains to you about the medicine. In addition to reinforcing what you need to know about the medication, it allows you to confirm that what was dispensed indeed is what your doctor prescribed. If there is any discrepancy, say so and ask for clarification. Ask how to pronounce the drug name (generic names are hard) to help avoid sound-alike and look-alike errors. "Metoprolol" can sound or look like "metformin" if you're not paying attention, for example.

When picking up a refill, it is good practice to open the bottle to make sure the tablets or capsules look the same as last month. If not, double check with the pharmacist or technician. It likely is the correct drug but a different generic manufacturer that month, but it is better to be safe and verify. Read the instruction label even if it is just a refill—your doctor might have made a change that you did not realize, or you might catch an error. As a rule, I always look at my prescription bottles before leaving the pharmacy to make sure I have the right prescription with my name on it. Finally, clarify any information, if needed, about how to take or monitor your medication at home. The more you know about your medications, the more you are empowered to take them correctly and recognize potential problems.

Denise's story illustrates how important it is to have basic information about your medications. The example is with insulin, which you might recognize is a medication considered high risk in older adults because of the potential to cause low blood sugar. Denise was prescribed short-acting insulin with instructions to take it "three times a day." Short-acting insulin works immediately to lower blood sugar and needs to be taken with meals to prevent blood sugar levels from falling too low. However, she did not recall this information and took her third dose at bedtime each day. As a result, she had woken up several nights with hypoglycemia and eventually was afraid to use her insulin at all. Once Denise was educated about the error, she no longer experienced hypoglycemia and had the confidence to take her insulin again, putting her diabetes control back on track.

GET A MEDICATION REVIEW ANNUALLY AND AT TRANSITIONS OF CARE

An annual medication review is like a regular car tune-up; it is good preventive care, but it also offers a way to defend against medication errors. Medication reviews are designed to identify medication-related problems, many of which also are medication errors. Many errors become evident only when there is an opportunity to speak with a pharmacist about when and how you take your medicines at home. In most cases, patients are unaware that they are causing a medication error, and a little extra education is all that is needed.

In addition, a medication review is a great time to make sure your medication list is free of any unnecessary drugs and that your daily schedule of when you take them is as simplified as possible. Take advantage of time with your pharmacist to review medication instructions and proper technique for inhalers and eye drops. Adherence errors might seem subtle but can be costly. The more you know about your medications and review this information, the more safeguards you have in place.

Any time you experience a transition of care, most notably when you return home from the hospital or a rehabilitation stay, a medication review is warranted. Before being discharged, a pharmacist or nurse should review your new medication list and compare it to what you were taking before.

Make sure any discrepancies are cleared up before you get home so you know what you should be taking and what should be stopped. A medication from home might be substituted for a similar drug in the hospital because of what is available in the hospital's pharmacy. This can lead to a duplication of therapy if you return home with the substituted medication from the hospital and also resume your pre-hospital medication. For example, if you were taking ramipril at home, but it was substituted for lisinopril in the hospital, you would not want to take both ramipril and lisinopril once you get back home.

Margaret provides a great example that illustrates the value of a medication review to uncover an error. She was taking her alendronate for osteoporosis once a week with lunch for over a year. Unfortunately, alendronate needs to be taken on an empty stomach only with water or the drug will not be absorbed. When her physician asked how things were going with the alendronate, she said she was taking it regularly and things were fine. The pharmacist saw no red flags because Margaret was getting the medicine refilled on time every month. Neither the physician nor the community pharmacist had reason to suspect a medication error for all these months. Margaret's error was only detectable when I asked her to describe in detail how she took each of her medicines. As a result of the error, Margaret wasted money on ineffective drug therapy plus lost a year of treatment. Her osteoporosis likely progressed, but at least she did not experience a fracture.

KEEP AN ACCURATE MEDICATION LIST

One of the risk factors for medication errors is physicians not knowing the patient's current medications. Thus, keeping a complete and accurate medication list is an important strategy. Tips for creating a medication list are summarized in **Box 15-1**. Remember that your medication list needs to include three categories of medications: prescription, over-the-counter, and dietary supplements. At minimum, list the drug name, dose, how many times a day you take it, and the reason you take it. Including when it was started and who prescribed it also can be helpful. The trick is to keep

Box 15-1. Ten Tips for Creating a Medication List
Keeping an accurate and complete medication list is without question one of the fundamental strategies to prevent medication errors, avoid unnecessary medications, and prevent adverse drug events. Here are the basic tips for creating your list.

1. Gather all of your current medications together. This needs to include all of your **prescription medicines, over-the-counter (OTC) products, and dietary supplements.** Don't forget to include vitamins and aspirin!
2. For each medication, write down the following:
   a. Name
   b. Strength (how many mg or mcg, for example)
   c. Dose, if you take more than just one tablet or capsule of that medicine; for example, "20 mg, two tablets at breakfast and dinner"
   d. How often you take it (how many times a day or per week, etc.)
   e. Special notes on how you take it (with or without food, thirty minutes before eating, etc.)
   f. Prescriber's name and roughly when it was started
3. Be sure to include topical products (creams, ointments, patches), injectable drugs, and drugs that are administered by your physician (for example, once monthly osteoporosis treatments)
4. Include medicines you take only sometimes ("as needed") at the bottom of your list.
5. List allergies and the type of reaction you had
6. Keep the list in your wallet or purse
7. Post the list on your refrigerator for emergency purposes
8. Share the list with close family members or friends
9. Bring the list with you to every doctor visit
10. Update the list as needed

the list current and have it available when you meet with members of your health-care team. Creating a list on your computer is an easy way to make changes and print an updated version when needed. You also can use an index card or download a template from the internet (more information is in Chapter 17, **Table 17-1** and **Figure 17-1**). If you have access to your medication list in your medical records through a patient portal, be sure to keep it updated.

DISPOSE OF OLD AND EXPIRED MEDICATIONS

One last tip to reduce the risk of medication errors is to dispose of medications you no longer use or that are expired. Having older medications in the house increases the risk of confusing an old prescription with your current medicines, for example. Mishaps can happen if a caregiver is assisting you or in an emergency situation. It is better to be safe than sorry. Safe disposal is important to reduce risks of accidental poisoning to children or pets, contamination of the water system, and drug diversion. Guidance on how to clean out your medicine cabinet and dispose of old medications is found in **Box 15-2** and in the Resources section.

SUMMARY

Although medication errors are widespread, by definition they are preventable. Individuals who are informed and engaged can help prevent errors by being part of the safety checks in the medication use process. Patient involvement is necessary to prevent errors in the home where the majority of medications are used. But patients can help catch errors during the prescribing, dispensing, and monitoring stages by consistently asking questions about their drug therapy. The various strategies and resources provided in this chapter empower patients to be vigilant to medication errors throughout the medication use process and during transitions of care.

Box 15-2. How to Clean Out Your Medicine Cabinet and Dispose of Old Medications

1. Identify nonprescription medicines that are expired.
   - Expiration dates are printed either on the label or directly on the bottle, usually on the bottom or near the neck. For creams or ointments, look on the crimp at the bottom of the tube.
   - A good rule of thumb for nonprescription products is to discard anything that is more than six months beyond the expiration date.

2. Identify prescription medications that are old, no longer used, or expired.
   - For prescription medicines, the expiration date is one year from the date it was filled at the pharmacy. This date is found on the printed pharmacy label.
   - If the medicine is in the original manufacturer's bottle, as with inhalers, eye drops, and some oral medications, use the manufacturer's expiration date found on the container as long as the medication has been stored properly.

3. Safely dispose of old and/or expired medications.
   - Combine all old prescription and nonprescription medications into a single bag and take them to a safe disposal (drug take-back) location. These sites incinerate the medications to minimize damage to the environment. Approved locations include most police stations and many pharmacies.
   - Do not flush tablets and capsules down the sink or toilet unless you are told to do so.
   - To dispose of medications at home, empty the pills into a bag, mix them with coffee grounds, cat litter, or another undesirable substance, seal it, and throw it in the trash.

What You Can Do at Home

- Know the generic names (and brand names, if applicable) of all your medications and why each is prescribed.
- Keep medications in their original containers; don't combine contents from different bottles, even if they are the same medicine. Each prescription label has important information on it.
- Keep a *complete* medication list that includes OTC products and dietary supplements.
- Take your medications as instructed every day; double check the medicine label to confirm that you've got the right drug and are taking it at the right time.
- Monitor for changes in how you feel day-to-day and for symptoms that might signal a side effect.
- Store your medications in one place.
- Properly dispose of old or expired medications (see Resources list).
- When transitioning from the hospital or another care setting to home, verify that you have the most current medication list; ask for "medication reconciliation"; make sure you know which medications to continue and which to stop.

What You Can Do with Your Pharmacist

- Use one pharmacy for all of your medications to maximize safeguards that reduce errors.
- Ask to speak with the pharmacist when you pick up your medicine; review the name, reason for use, instructions, side effects, and interactions; make sure instructions are clear.
- Ask about monitoring that you can do at home to reduce risk of an adverse event; know what side effects to look for and what to do if they occur.

- If you are told to split a tablet, check with the pharmacist to make sure it is scored, meaning it has a line or indent down the middle. Purchase a tablet splitter.
- Ask the pharmacist for advice on how to simplify your drug regimen.
- Review proper administration technique for inhalers, eye drops, injectables, and patches.
- Take notes or get information in writing.
- Make sure you have the correct medications before leaving the pharmacy.
- Get an annual medication review.

What You Can Do with Your Physician

- Keep a complete and accurate medication list that you share with all of your physicians.
- Have each physician review your medication list before prescribing a medication or making changes.
- Make sure each physician knows your drug allergies and previous adverse drug reactions.
- Have the physician tell you the name and strength of a new medication and why it is prescribed; use this information as a double check at the pharmacy when you pick it up.
- Ask for information on the risks and benefits of a new medication in terms you understand. Remember that fewer medications are safer and reduce the risk of an error.
- Take notes; bring along a trusted family member or friend as a backup.
- Follow medical advice if you are asked to make changes to your medications (for example, starting or stopping a medication or adjusting the amount you take).
- Communicate concerns or questions about your medications or health conditions; if you hear different things from different physicians, ask for clarification.

RESOURCES

Safe Medication Use

- ConsumerMedSafety for Older Adults by the Institute for
  Safe Medication Practices:
  - https://www.consumermedsafety.org/safety-tips
    /medicine-in-older-adults
- Centers for Disease Control and Prevention (CDC)
  Medication Safety Program:
  - https://www.cdc.gov/medicationsafety/index.html
- Taking Medications, Agency for Healthcare Research and
  Quality:
  - https://www.ahrq.gov/patients-consumers/diagnosis
    -treatment/treatments/index.html
- Safe use of medication for older adults, National Institute on
  Aging:
  - https://www.nia.nih.gov/health
    /safe-use-medicines-older-adults
- World Health Organization, 5 Moments for Medical Safety
  (downloadable brochure of questions to ask):
  - https://www.who.int/publications/i/item/WHO
    -HIS-SDS-2019.4 or https://www.who.int/initiatives
    /medication-without-harm

Medication Error Reporting Programs
- FDA MedWatch program: https://www.fda.gov/safety
  /medwatch-fda-safety-information-and-adverse-event
  -reporting-program
- Institute of Safe Medication Practices consumer website:
  https://www.consumermedsafety.org/

How to Dispose of Old and Expired Medications

- Safe Pharmacy by National Association of Boards of Pharmacy, find a drug disposal site near you: https://safe.pharmacy/
- Where and how to dispose of unused medicine: https://www.fda.gov/consumers/consumer-updates /where-and-how-dispose-unused-medicines
- Script Your Future, safe drug disposal, where and how: https://scriptyourfuture.org/health-conditions /safe-drug-disposal/

Chapter 16

Avoid Medication Overload and Inappropriate Polypharmacy

Optimizing medication use means finding the right combination of medications at the right dosages and for the correct duration of use for a specific patient. It involves addressing both over- and underuse of medications and inappropriate prescribing. This chapter focuses on strategies to reduce medication overload and inappropriate polypharmacy. These concepts were discussed in Chapter 4 and refer to the use of medications that are not needed, not effective, or associated with harms that are greater than benefits. Thus, this chapter speaks to the heart of this book, which is to use medications more safely and avoid unnecessary and harmful drug therapy. Patients need to be empowered to be part of not just the prescribing process, but also deprescribing medications when appropriate. Starting a medication does not necessarily mean you have to take it for the rest of your life. The challenge for you now is to actively participate with your health-care team to agree upon what drug therapy is truly necessary for you and which medications represent overload.

SLOW DOWN THE URGE TO PRESCRIBE

Prescribing medications is best approached in a thoughtful, more cautious manner in older adults. As long as your health is stable, be willing to pause and respectfully question the value of adding another drug. It is okay to be skeptical about a recommended medication until you get more information. Of course, in an emergency situation, these comments do not apply. But in many non-emergent situations, less can be more. A hard lesson we have learned regarding polypharmacy is that it is difficult to stop medications once they are started. Patients have often observed that it is easy for their doctors to add a new medication, but they are far less willing to stop one. Therefore, take time to explore both drug and non-drug therapy options before making a decision to start a long-term medication.

In addition, goals of drug therapy need to be individualized throughout a patient's health journey. For example, goals for managing diabetes and blood pressure should be reassessed over time, as circumstances likely will change. Therapy that was appropriate at age fifty may lead to adverse outcomes at age seventy-five. To illustrate this point, an appropriately aggressive goal when treating diabetes usually is a hemoglobin A1c goal of less than 7 percent in adults who are younger and with few health conditions. However, a more flexible goal of less than 7.5 percent or 8 percent might be appropriate in an older individual, depending on multiple health conditions, risk of low blood sugar, and patient preferences, for example.[319]

Strive to take only medications that are truly necessary based on information you and your physician have discussed and after you have evaluated your options. **Box 16-1** lists questions that can help you and your physician discuss risks and benefits when a new medicine is being considered. Shared decision making needs to incorporate your preferences and can help limit excessive prescribing. Listen to sound advice, of course; but ultimately, you need to be comfortable with drug therapy decisions and willing to follow the treatment plan.

Box 16-1. Questions to Help Assess Risk and Benefit of a Medication

1. What is the reason or the clinical indication for prescribing this medication?
2. How effective is this medication for treating the condition?
   - For example, in the clinical studies, did it work in 90 percent of patients or only 40 percent? How clinically meaningful was the effect? Some medications offer only marginal clinical benefit, even though the measured outcome of the drug was "statistically significant" in the studies. For example, shortening the time to get to sleep by eighteen minutes may not be worth the risk of a fall-related injury or memory impairment.[320]
3. What risks are associated with the medication?
   - Risks include not only side effects, but cost and added pill burden, for example. As part of shared decision making, talk with your physician about risks and benefits. But you need to have access to accurate, reliable, and complete information. A friend, social media, or the internet may not be your best source.
4. How and when does the medication have to be taken?
   - Consider how easy or difficult it might be for you to adhere to the medication instructions or to administer it (if it is an injectable or an inhaled medicine, for example).
5. How long will it take to see the benefit of the medication?
   - You might see a benefit immediately or within days, as with treating pain or reflux disease. Or the benefit might take weeks, which is the case when starting an antidepressant; months, as with glucosamine-chondroitin to treat osteoarthritis; or even years, as with drug therapy

for osteoporosis. Are you willing to take a medication regularly, even if there is a delay in the onset of a noticeable effect or long-term clinical benefit?

6. Is there a non-drug option that is known to be effective? How does it compare with the non-drug option(s)?

AVOID THE PRESCRIBING CASCADE

Too often, a new medication is the answer when a new symptom arises. Instead, one of the first questions that should be asked is, "Could one of the medications I already take be causing the new symptom?" Adverse drug reactions can mimic a new condition, which can lead to a prescribing cascade. This term was first introduced in Chapter 5. Thus, any time a new symptom arises, medications should be suspected until proven otherwise. Before a medication is added, be sure your physician has evaluated if the symptom might actually be caused by an existing medication you are taking. **Table 16-1** lists a handful of common adverse drug reactions that can look like other health conditions and lead to a prescribing cascade. Myriad other examples exist, of course. In some cases, a prescribing cascade might be the best treatment approach and thus adding a medication would be appropriate.

Make sure your physicians have access to a list that contains *all* of the medications you take—including nonprescription products. As discussed in Chapter 6, dietary supplements and OTC products can cause side effects and drug interactions, too. Your pharmacist is often easier to access in between doctor visits and is a great resource to review your medications for possible side effects that can be causing a new symptom.

A recent study by Barbara Farrell and colleagues confirms the challenges involved in identifying a prescribing cascade.[321] One of these challenges is that clinicians and patients are unaware of the types of side effects that medications can cause. The study highlighted the opportunity for patients to help prevent prescribing cascades by knowing their medications sufficiently, including possible side effects. In this way, individuals can be proactive and monitor for symptoms that could be a medication side

Table 16-1. Examples of Adverse Drug Reactions that Can Mimic Health Conditions

Adverse drug reaction	Examples of medications that can cause the reaction (lists are not complete)
Confusion, decreased cognitive function	• amitriptyline • diphenhydramine • olanzapine • oxybutynin
Constipation	• diltiazem, verapamil • opioid pain medications
Increased blood pressure	• nonsteroidal anti-inflammatory drugs (NSAIDs)
Insomnia, difficulty sleeping	• alcohol • bupropion • caffeine • pseudoephedrine
Urinary incontinence	• alcohol • donepezil • doxazosin (in women) • furosemide

effect. Farrell and colleagues conclude that both clinicians and patients need to be more knowledgeable about medication side effects and routinely question if new symptoms or a worsening medical condition could be caused by a drug. In addition, they need to be willing to re-evaluate the benefits and risks of a drug therapy and discuss the possibility of reducing or stopping a medication before adding another one.

FOCUS ON NONDRUG TREATMENT OPTIONS

Investing in healthy lifestyle changes and nondrug treatment strategies that have evidence to support their effectiveness in managing specific health conditions is one of the most basic ways to avoid adding a medication to your regimen. When faced with a new diagnosis, a great question to ask is whether there are nondrug approaches that can be tried first to manage the condition. However, these options often get overlooked. Our health culture leans toward prescribing rather than the more time-intensive process of educating patients about nondrug options. I've seen patients tell their doctors they have pain and receive a prescription for a muscle relaxer that has no benefit and significant side effects, rather than be told about ways to use heat, ice, or exercise to address the issue.

The benefits of healthy lifestyle choices were highlighted in Chapter 7 as a way to delay or even avoid the need for drug therapy for some diagnoses. For other conditions, short-term therapy can be helpful but should not be continued long-term (chronically), such as with gastroesophageal reflux disease (GERD) and insomnia. In these cases, nondrug strategies can be instrumental to improve symptoms and quality of life. Once drug therapy is started, though, this does not mean you have a free pass on healthy lifestyle behaviors; you still need to continue good nutrition, physical activity, and other healthy modifications to maximize health outcomes.

KNOW THE GOALS OF DRUG THERAPY

Know the goals for each medication you are prescribed. What is it treating and how will you know if it is working? What side effects can you watch for? How long do you need to take it to tell if it is effective? When a medication is started, you should know the reason—the goal—and how you will know when that goal is met. Examples of goals of therapy include relief of a particular symptom or a blood level that returns to a normal range. Other goals are short-term markers that indicate long-term benefits, such as with blood pressure control and hemoglobin A1c level.

If the goal is reached—for example, your blood pressure is less than 130/80 mmHg, or your depression symptoms have improved—then therapy should be continued to maintain the good effect. Sometimes the dose of a medication can be reduced once the initial goal is reached. Therefore, it can be helpful to check with your doctor or pharmacist to ensure you are taking the lowest effective dose for long-term therapy.

On the other hand, if the goal is not reached, it is important to first confirm that you were taking the medication properly, the dose was sufficient (therapeutic), and you took it for a long-enough duration that the drug had time to be effective. It also is important to confirm that the right drug was chosen to treat the condition. If everything listed is in order, then the next step might be to add another medication (intensify therapy), as when treating high blood pressure. But if the goal was to treat a specific symptom (such as pain or stomach acid reflux) and this goal was not met, the best option more likely is to stop the drug and figure out another approach. In some cases, an ineffective drug can mean that the diagnosis is incorrect and different drug treatment is warranted. Several times I have seen patients who were started on a medicine to treat "stomach pain," but did not have improvement in symptoms months later. In these situations, the diagnosis and medication need to be reevaluated.

Micah's story illustrates the importance of knowing the goals of therapy. Micah was a seventy-nine-year-old gentleman who had joint pain in his hand, shoulder, and hip and was diagnosed with gout by his primary care physician. The doctor prescribed a one-week course of prednisone for the immediate pain and inflammation plus allopurinol to be continued daily. The pain resolved but subsequently returned when the prednisone was stopped. A month later, Micah called his doctor and told him the pain was still bothersome. The doctor prescribed a second one-week course of prednisone. Again, Micah felt better for the week, but the symptoms returned. This continued for a few more months. He was on the right treatment for gout, but the pattern of Micah's symptoms and lack of response raised suspicion that maybe it was not the right diagnosis. I encouraged Micah to contact his doctor to reassess his situation.

In the end, it was not gout. Micah ended up seeing a rheumatologist who diagnosed his pain in multiple joints as another inflammatory condition (polymyalgia rheumatica). Allopurinol was stopped, and Micah was initiated on appropriate—and effective—drug therapy.

USE ONE DRUG TO TREAT TWO CONDITIONS

Many medications can be used to treat more than one health condition. Although not extremely commonplace, using one drug to treat two conditions is another strategy for limiting polypharmacy. Examples include prescribing duloxetine to treat depression and pain, or doxazosin to treat high blood pressure and symptoms of an enlarged prostate. The best way to find out if this strategy is an option for you is to ask your pharmacist or physician. This is a great question that can be part of an annual medication review. Sometimes a dual-treatment medication is simply overlooked, or maybe it already has been considered for you but is not an option based on your medical information.

IDENTIFY MEDICATIONS THAT CAN BE DEPRESCRIBED

Deprescribing is the official term for discontinuing or reducing dosages of medications and was introduced in Chapter 4. Interest in deprescribing has blossomed in recent years in response to the growing concerns surrounding inappropriate polypharmacy. Medications that no longer are needed or no longer helpful should be stopped. Prescribing inertia refers to the process of continuing medications year after year without questioning whether they still truly are necessary. Thus, it is okay to ask your physician to critically look at your medications and question if any can be stopped or reduced—including your nonprescription drugs.

Your body and how it reacts to medications can change over time. Thus, medications that once were helpful may no longer be needed or could be contributing to a side effect that looks like "getting old." In some cases, the reason a drug was first prescribed might have resolved, or you might simply need less intense therapy as your body and overall health has changed. The balance of benefit and harm can shift as we get older, making some medications potentially inappropriate for older individuals. As the number of people living into their nineties and past a hundred years of age increases, there is an urgent need to better understand which drug therapy is still safe and beneficial and which drug therapy might be higher risk and should be stopped.

Have a pharmacist review all of your medications for opportunities to deprescribe. It sometimes can be hard for physicians to recognize opportunities to stop or reduce medications. In the absence of obvious concerns, prescribers have little reason to question your current drug therapy and likely are more focused on other health issues you might have. Thus, the expertise and outside perspective of a pharmacist can be valuable to identify potentially unnecessary or ineffective medications. The value of a medication review and suggestions on how to obtain one were provided in Chapter 3.

Be willing to listen to recommendations about stopping medications that may no longer be safe or effective, even if you are hesitant to discontinue them. I have spoken with many clients who insist they don't want to stop a high-risk medication. Remember that medications have tradeoffs.

A final word of caution is that if a medication is identified as one that can be stopped, be careful to confirm the best way to stop it. Certain medications cannot be stopped abruptly, but need to gradually be reduced over time based on the health condition being treated and the potential for drug withdrawal symptoms. This applies to drugs that treat cardiovascular conditions and seizures, and drug classes like antidepressants, benzodiazepines, and opioid pain medications, among others. When in doubt, it is safer to slowly reduce the medication rather than stop it all at once; check with your physician or pharmacist. And never stop a medication on your own; always discuss it with your physician or pharmacist first.

UTILIZE RESOURCES TO START THE CONVERSATION

There are two resources that are medical-expert approved and intended to promote conversations between patients and physicians about drug therapy. The first resource is the AGS Beers Criteria, a list of potentially inappropriate medications (PIMs) that was discussed in Chapter 10.[322] PIMs are identified by geriatrics experts as higher-risk drugs in older adults and are recommended to be avoided when possible. Safer alternatives tend to be available in most situations. Thus, inquiring about PIMs, namely drugs that are included on the AGS Beers Criteria, is a way to start a conversation about possible medications that could be deprescribed.

Keep in mind that PIMs are *potentially* inappropriate and not *definitely* inappropriate. Sometimes they are the most appropriate option. In these cases, make sure you are taking the lowest effective dose and that you and your doctor are being mindful to watch for any unwanted effects.

The second resource is the Choosing Wisely campaign.[323] This national program was created in 2012 to reduce overuse in health care by identifying low-value care. The goal is to spur conversations between patients and physicians about tests, procedures, or treatments that should be questioned. Over eighty medical specialty groups have developed lists that are accessible on the Choosing Wisely website (www.choosingwisely .org). Among these eighty specialty groups are two lists from professional pharmacy associations that focus solely on medication practices that should be questioned. Examples of items from the Choosing Wisely lists developed by these two associations and the American Geriatrics Society are provided in **Table 16-2**. The American Society of Consultant Pharmacists is a professional association that represents pharmacists and other health-care professionals who serve older adults. Thus, its list contains ten medication-related items that are all specific to older adults. Although the Choosing Wisely website is intended for clinicians, community organizations, and employers to promote to consumers, anyone is able to search, download, and print out topics of interest to discuss with their physicians.

Table 16-2. Selected Medication-Related Items from *Choosing Wisely*

Medical specialty association	Sample items of "Things Clinicians and Patients Should Question"
The American Geriatrics Society	• Don't use benzodiazepines or other sedative-hypnotics in older adults as first choice for insomnia, agitation, or delirium. • Don't prescribe a medication without conducting a drug regimen review.
American Society of Consultant Pharmacists	• Don't initiate medications to treat new and emerging symptoms without first ascertaining that the new symptom is not an adverse drug event of an already prescribed medication. • Don't recommend highly anticholinergic medications in older adults without first considering safer alternatives or non-drug measures.
American Society of Health-system Pharmacists	• Do not prescribe or indefinitely continue medications for patients on five or more medications, without a comprehensive medication review, including prescription and over-the-counter medications and dietary supplements, to determine whether any of the medications or supplements can be discontinued and assure all medications to be taken by the patient are optimized for the patient's specific medical and social conditions. • Do not prescribe patients medications during care transitions (such as hospital discharge) without verifying that all medications have an indication and are still needed, and that discharge medications will not result in duplication, drug interactions, or adverse events.

SUMMARY

Inappropriate polypharmacy and medication overload are terms that embody the problem of excessive medication use. However you wish to name the problem, it is a massive issue that permeates our health-care system and requires an all-hands-on-deck approach. The solution clearly requires patient involvement. This chapter presented strategies to empower patients to bring up conversations with their health-care team, utilize the expertise of a geriatric pharmacist, and advocate for medication use that is limited to drug therapy that is truly needed and beneficial.

What You Can Do at Home

- Keep a complete medication list as described in Chapter 15 (see **Box 15-1**).
- Read all medication labels to ensure good adherence (right drug, right time, etc.).
- Read all medication labels to avoid drug interactions at home, such as with food, alcohol, or nonprescription products.
- Use one pharmacy to fill your prescriptions so that a pharmacist can screen for interactions and view all your prescribed medications.
- Avoid combination OTC products; choose products to treat just the symptoms you have.
- Follow through on nondrug strategies when applicable as a way to manage your health conditions and the need for added drug therapy.

What You Can Do with Your Pharmacist

- Confirm that any new medications do not have important interactions or duplicate current therapy.

- Ask for a review to identify medications that could be a part of a prescribing cascade.
- Confirm you have chosen correct OTC products or dietary supplements that will be safe and effective for your symptoms; choose single-ingredient products when possible.
- Ask if you are taking any medications that are considered potentially inappropriate for older adults.
- Get an annual medication review with special attention to unnecessary or ineffective medications that could be discontinued.
- Make sure old and discontinued medications are marked inactive in your pharmacy's computer profile, especially if you are enrolled in an automatic refill program.
- Discuss goals of therapy for your medications and how you can monitor for these goals at home.

What You Can Do with Your Physician

- Have your medication list with you at every office visit and make sure the prescriber reviews it before adding a new medication.
- Slow down prescribing; ask if there still is a valid reason for taking each medication and if any can be reduced or discontinued (deprescribed).
- Ask if one drug can be used to treat two conditions to avoid adding a separate medication.
- Ask about nondrug strategies to improve your health and as alternatives to drug therapy.
- Let your primary care physician know when a specialist wants to start a new medication (and vice versa); advocate for your physicians to coordinate your care with each other.
- Discuss risks and benefits of any medications that your physician is considering.

- Agree on goals of therapy for each medication and regularly review if those goals are met; discuss opportunities to adjust drug therapy based on reaching or not reaching those goals.
- For any medications that will be stopped, develop a plan for how to do so safely and monitor for symptoms.
- Use the AGS Beers Criteria and Choosing Wisely lists to help start a conversation about potentially unnecessary or harmful drug therapy.

RESOURCES

- BeMedWise: http://bemedwise.org/
  o Encourages communication about medications between patients and health-care professionals; has multiple printable handouts and other resources about medication safety
- Choosing Wisely Campaign: http://www.choosingwisely.org/
  o Created by the American Board of Internal Medicine Foundation. Provides lists by medical and pharmacy specialty groups to increase conversation between physicians and patients about treatments—including drug therapy—that should be questioned.
- Health In Aging: https://www.healthinaging.org/
  o Created by the American Geriatrics Society. Contains several resources about medication use and older adults.
- World Health Organization, 5 Moments for Medical Safety (downloadable brochure of questions to ask): https://www .who.int/publications/i/item/WHO-HIS-SDS-2019.4 or https://www.who.int/initiatives/medication-without-harm

CHAPTER 17

Take Medications as Instructed

There are numerous factors that affect a person's ability to adhere to their medication regimen. Medication adherence was defined in Chapter 8 as the extent to which individuals take their medications according to the instructions provided by health-care professionals. Taking medications—and taking them correctly—is necessary to achieve desired outcomes of drug therapy. Medications not taken cannot be effective. Yet adherence remains problematic for many older individuals for a variety of reasons that range from cost to side effects to forgetfulness. On the other hand, there are many people for whom adherence is not a problem. Their medication regimens have become routine, and they take their medications like clockwork. Each person's situation is unique, and subsequently, the approach to improving medication adherence must be tailored to the individual. Efforts to address barriers are most effective when tackled jointly by the patient and health-care team. Ultimately, you are the consumer and the person responsible for taking your medications on a regular basis. For most individuals, this means every day. Armed with an awareness of the scope of the problem, you now have the opportunity to be more proactive in managing your medication regimen at home so you can take them in the correct manner. This chapter provides tips and strategies to address some of the more common adherence barriers.

Before we jump into talking about adherence strategies, there are two considerations that will make adherence easier for you from the outset. The first is that ideally you are taking only what is truly of benefit for your health. Your medication list should be free of unnecessary and ineffective medications that merely increase the burden of how many you have to take every day. The second consideration is that ideally you should believe in the value of your medicines. If you have doubts about whether you need a medication, for example, you likely will feel less motivated to take it. Previous chapters have talked about ways to work with your physician and pharmacist to reduce unnecessary medications. If you have questions about how your medications are helping you, seek answers from your health-care team. Once you have your medication list together and you are committed to taking the medicines on that list properly, we can turn to strategies to support good adherence.

BE INFORMED

Having basic information about your medications is key to taking them properly. At the very least, know why the medicines are prescribed, how you are supposed to take each one, and what the common side effects are. Ideally, know all eight essential items from Chapter 14. It might sound basic, but take a minute to read the instructions on the label, even if you have been taking it for a long time. I have seen too many examples of clients who made adherence errors with medications they had been taking for years because they relied on what they thought were the correct instructions but never bothered to carefully reread the label. For many individuals, nonadherence is unintentional; people just are not aware of the mistake.

Make sure you know enough about your health conditions to understand the role of the medications in treating those conditions. Will the drug work quickly or is there a lag time before it takes effect? What are possible risks if you forget to take a dose of the medicine? If instructions are to take a medicine "as needed," be sure you know what symptoms the drug is supposed to treat so you know when you should take it, as these types of medications are not taken on a regular schedule. These are just a few of many questions that can help you better understand the role and value of the medications you are prescribed.

Finally, ask for information in writing. If you are not familiar with a medical term, have your clinician write it down for you. If something is not clear, ask for it to be repeated or explained in a different way. It's always a good idea to have a friend or family member with you as a second set of eyes and ears and to help take notes.

KEEP A REGULAR SCHEDULE FOR TAKING YOUR MEDICATIONS

Develop a schedule for taking your medications, and stick with it every day. The schedule should fit in with your daily activities and become something you do as a matter of routine, like getting dressed and brushing your teeth. Taking medications "whenever I think of it" is not a good answer, but one I often hear. Breakfast, lunch, dinner, and bedtime are the four standard times around which most medications can be scheduled. Some individuals might schedule a dosing time when their favorite nightly television show is on, and this can work, too, as long as it happens every day to serve as a cue to take your medicines. Everyone should write out their medication schedule with the specific times that each medication needs to be taken; this and other reminder aids are discussed soon.

SIMPLIFY YOUR DRUG REGIMEN

When figuring out the best routine for taking your daily medications (and even your weekly or monthly ones), first work with your pharmacist to simplify your medication schedule. Your medications should not end up ruling your day; they should fit into a schedule that works for you and your activities. Ideally, you should be able to limit the number of times each day that you have to interrupt an activity just to take a medication. A regimen where medications have to be taken only once- or twice-daily would be ideal, but may not be possible. Your pharmacist can guide you on how to safely group medications together so that the schedule for how often you have to take medications is manageable and fits into your daily activities. In addition, your pharmacist can make recommendations to your physician to switch to once-daily options or combination pills when available. This also is a good time for your pharmacist to review your regimen for any unnecessary medications that might be stopped, including nonprescription products you take regularly.

USE REMINDER AIDS

Difficulty remembering to take medications is one of the most common reasons for poor adherence. That is why it is so important to establish a routine schedule and make sure it is as simplified as possible. Even so, forgetfulness can rear its ugly head. In addition, a growing number of older adults are aging at home with some degree of memory loss or cognitive impairment. For these individuals, it is important to have family members or other caregivers involved to support adherence and have reminder aids in place.

There is an abundance of different kinds of memory aids and reminder tools available, from paper calendars and pill organizers to smart caps and smartphone calendar reminders. The simplest tool is a written or printed medication list that indicates the specific time of day that each medication is given. For individuals who take multiple medications, a printed schedule is essential. Posting it on the refrigerator where it can be accessed in an emergency is recommended. Templates of medication lists are available online or you can create your own version. An example of a medication list template is provided in **Figure 17-1**.

Name: _Honey Clover_ Date of birth: _5/16/34_ Date: _5/5/22; 1/18/23_

Name of medicine	Strength	What is this medicine for?	How much do I use and how often?	Prescriber	Date started
Valsartan (Diovan)	160 mg	High blood pressure	1 tablet once daily in morning	Dr. Jones	7/31/2018
Atorvastatin (Lipitor)	20 mg	High cholesterol	1 tablet once daily in morning	Dr. Jones	5/5/2022
Gabapentin (Neurontin)	300 mg	Nerve pain in feet	2 tablets in morning, 1 tablet at noon, 2 tablets at bedtime	Dr. Smith	Dose increased 1/18/2023
Vitamin D	1000 units	Replace low vitamin D levels	1 tablet daily at bedtime	Dr. Smith	1/18/2023

Figure 17-1. Example of a Medication List Template

One of the least expensive and must functional tools is a pill organizer that can be filled in advance for the week. It is a great way to remind individuals if they took their medications already, as the slot in the organizer will be empty if the pills for that dosing time already were taken. This helps to avoid errors of doubling up on a dose, for example, in case the person cannot recall. Pill organizers come in small and large sizes to hold different amounts of pills. They also come with different numbers of slots per day to handle regimens ranging most commonly from once- to four-times daily, but can be found with up to seven slots per day. Most accommodate just one week's supply of medications; however, fancier versions are available that can be filled for up to a month. Be mindful that not all medications can be placed in the pill organizer. Some may need to be kept in original packaging; others like eye drops, inhalers, and injectable medicines need to be stored separately. Finally, it is not appropriate to fill "as needed" medicines in the pill organizer, as they are not taken on a scheduled basis.

There are a number of reminder aids that provide alarms or other notifications to take medication doses throughout the day. These include watches, pagers, and medication alarm clocks. Smart phones can be programmed with reminders, as well. Adding a calendar reminder can be helpful, particularly for medications taken once a week or once a month. Use of smart phone applications (apps) is another resource of growing interest in the digital age; however, as with many medical apps, you need to approach these with eyes wide open. Over 2,000 medication adherence apps are available for both Android and Apple operating platforms.[324,325] These apps are of variable quality and functionality. Not all are well-suited for complex drug regimens (multiple medications needing to be taken multiple times per day), and none have been studied yet to evaluate if they can help with long-term adherence for patients with chronic health conditions. In 2021, Claudine Backes and colleagues evaluated four free and three paid apps from both the scientific and patient perspectives.[326] They found that none of the apps were of high quality. Patients interested in using adherence apps should consider cost, security, and how they protect personal information.

Multi-dose packaging is available through many pharmacies as a way to help with adherence, namely strip or pouch packaging and blister cards. With these packaging services, your different prescriptions are pre-sorted by the day and time the medications need to be taken. For example, all of the 8 a.m. pills would be in one pouch or blister bubble and all 5 p.m. pills would be in another. You then need to simply either tear off the next pouch on the strip of medications or punch them out from a blister card. If you are interested in this type of adherence packaging for yourself or someone you are caring for, ask if your local pharmacy offers adherence packaging or if the pharmacist can recommend another way to access this type of packaging.

Finally, fancier electronic dispensing machines can be filled for up to ninety days at a time. These more expensive tools can be a great asset for individuals who need a little more assistance with managing their medications but are still living independently. Caregivers can monitor the devices remotely using a smart phone app, for example. Some of the features to consider when choosing a dispensing machine include how many medications the device can hold and how many doses each day it can handle; how often the device needs to be refilled; whether it can be locked; and what type of alarms it offers—for example, visual or auditory.[327]

A summary of various adherence aids is provided in **Table 17-1.** The list is not intended to be exhaustive, but to shed some light on the variety of options available. Consult with your pharmacist ways to apply these or other strategies to a reminder system that works best for you.

Table 17-1. Medication Adherence Reminder Aids

Type of reminder aid	Examples or sources
Printed medication list templates	• Agency for Healthcare Research and Quality: "My Medicines List," https://www.ahrq.gov/sites/default/files/wysiwyg/health-literacy/my-medicines-list.pdf • American Society of Consultant Pharmacists: "Personal Medication List," https://www.ascp.com/mpage/factsheets • Food and Drug Administration: "My Medicine Record," https://www.fda.gov/drugs/resources-you-drugs/my-medicine-record • *Others available by searching for medication list templates*

Pill organizers	• e-pill Medication Reminders, https://www.epill.com/, has organizers with slots for up to seven times per day, monthly pill organizers, plus many other unique aids
Alarm reminder resources	• Available from multiple retail and online locations • Medication timer caps for prescription bottles • Alarm watches (e.g., Cadex), personalized talking alarm clocks (e.g., MedCenter®)
Electronic dispensing machines	• Many brands are available: EMMA (Electronic Medication Management Assistant), Hero, Karie, Livi, MedTime, and Philips Medication Dispenser, to name a few
Other resources (check with your community pharmacy)	• Multi-dose packaging, blister packaging • Medication synchronization • Pharmacy-generated reminders

GET YOUR MEDICATIONS REFILLED ON TIME

To avoid gaps in drug therapy if you run out of a medication, it is a good habit to call the pharmacy when you have five to seven days remaining of your medication. Don't wait until the day before you need the refill. The pharmacy needs time to not just fill the prescription, but to make sure it is in stock or to contact your doctor's office if a new prescription is needed. Pharmacists work hard to minimize the impact of drug shortages and supply chain problems, so avoiding last minute refill requests is helpful.

If you struggle to get medications refilled on time because your medications have different dates that they need to be refilled, talk with your pharmacist about ways to correct this. A unique tool that some pharmacies offer is called "medication synchronization." This is a program that aligns the refill dates of your prescriptions so that they can be picked up on the same day each month. There are several benefits of "med sync" programs, the first of which is the need for fewer trips to the pharmacy to pick up refills (or fewer deliveries if you have your medications delivered). By having a coordinated date on which you can pick up multiple refills, it reduces the risk that you will be late with a refill, thereby avoiding gaps in your therapy. It also provides for an additional touch point with the pharmacist on a monthly basis to check on how things are going at home with your medications. Ask your pharmacist if you are eligible for medication synchronization to coordinate refill dates for your long-term medications.

Enrolling in an automatic refill program with your pharmacy is promoted as another way to ensure timely medication refills. This can work well for many individuals. There also are drawbacks to these programs that can make them less-than-ideal. One concern is that it can lead to dispensing errors if a physician discontinues a medication but does not convey this update to the pharmacy. The pharmacy unknowingly would then still automatically refill the stopped medication, and the patient can end up continuing it in error. I've also seen situations where my clients used the pharmacy's automatic refill program and the delivery service and ended up with months' worth of unused prescriptions at home because the pharmacy kept refilling and delivering them every month, even though the medicines were not being used routinely.

KNOW PROPER TECHNIQUE FOR ADMINISTERING SPECIAL DOSAGE FORMS

Make sure you know the proper technique for any of your non-oral medications. Mistakes are common when using inhalers and eye drops, which are some of the more widely used non-oral products. Inhalers are used to treat chronic obstructive pulmonary disease (COPD) or asthma, and eye drops are the most common way to manage conditions like glaucoma. Improper technique can lead to poor symptom control and disease progression.

In the case of inhalers, poor technique is a frequent contributor to exacerbations of COPD and the need for hospitalization. Therefore, making sure you use the correct technique with your inhalers is critical. There currently is an array of inhaler devices available, each with a unique series of steps for proper administration. If you use an inhaler, it is important to understand how to set up the inhaler and what kind of in-breath (inhalation) is needed; for example, slow and steady or sharp and quick. Review your inhaler technique periodically (as part of your annual medication review, for example) with one of your health-care professionals. If needed, be proactive and ask someone to review your technique to be sure.

Eye drop technique also is prone to errors. There is a series of steps that need to be followed to ensure the drug effectively gets into the eye. Aiming the drop so it lands in the eye and then closing the eye for at least one minute are part of proper technique. Two adherence aids can be used when needed: an eye drop guide can help aim the drop, and an eye drop squeezer can help patients who have difficulty squeezing the bottle. If you use more than one medicine, you need to know to separate each medicine by five minutes to allow each drop to get absorbed. One of my clients applied his two glaucoma eye drop medications one right after the other, which led to neither drug being fully effective. Another client I worked with blinked away her eye drop and let it run down her cheek.

KEEP YOUR MEDICATIONS AFFORDABLE

High cost is a barrier for many older adults and an ongoing public health concern. When financial burdens interfere with you taking your medications, speak with your physician and pharmacist right away. Ask about lower cost generic options if you are prescribed a brand-name drug. Options include switching to the generic version of the brand-name product or to a generic version of a therapeutic alternative (a closely related drug, often from the same drug class) that will have the same clinical effect. There also might be private or government-funded programs for which you qualify to help reduce costs. Do not assume that your prescriber knows what your co-pay is for a medication or how much you are willing or able to pay. Your pharmacist and physician are on your side and can help you navigate these challenges and find an affordable regimen for you. Tips and resources to help make your medications more affordable are provided in **Box 17-1**. Talk with your pharmacist and physician about the suggestions on this list. It is not exhaustive and some ideas might be better options for you than others.

Box 17-1. Tips and Resources to Reduce Medication Costs

- Ask your pharmacist and physician about generic and lower-cost therapeutic alternatives that are equally effective.
- Ask your pharmacist if it will be less expensive to get a ninety-day supply (rather than thirty-day) for long-term medications.
- Ask your pharmacist if tablet-splitting is an option for any of your medications.
- Find out from your insurance plan if a similar medication has a lower co-pay; if yes, ask your physician if switching is an option.
- Ask for a medication review to eliminate overlapping or unnecessary medications, identify drugs that could be part of a prescribing cascade, and eliminate OTC drugs and dietary supplements that duplicate other therapy or are of low clinical benefit.
- Ask if your pharmacy has a drug discount program.
- Take your medications as instructed (be adherent); stretching out medications to make them last longer can be more expensive in the long run.
- Maximize nondrug strategies that are proven to be effective for managing some of your health conditions.
- Explore state assistance programs and get local Medicare help with one-on-one counseling.
    - State Health Insurance Assistance Programs: https://www.shiphelp.org/
- Find out about patient assistance programs by drug manufacturers.
    - RxAssist: https://www.rxassist.org/
    - NeedyMeds: https://www.needymeds.org/ (plus other cost-saving resources)
    - Medicine Assistance Tool: https://medicineassistancetool.org/

- Use BenefitsCheckUp®, a free online tool by the National Council on Aging (NCOA); it provides an individualized report of public and private programs to lower costs for older adults: https://benefitscheckup.org/
- Take advantage of the Medicare Part D annual re-enrollment period to find the best plan for the coming year.
- Find out if you qualify for Extra Help from Medicare Part D: https://www.medicare.gov/ or https://benefitscheckup.org/

Importantly, if you are enrolled in a Medicare Part D plan, be sure to take advantage of the annual re-enrollment period to review your plan options every year. Part D plans can change formularies (preferred drug lists). What worked for you the current year might not be your cheapest option for the next year.

As emphasized throughout this book, make sure you are not taking unnecessary medications, including nonprescription products and drugs involved in a prescribing cascade. Dietary supplements can be pricey and many offer limited or no benefit. Get an annual medication review to identify these low-value supplements that can be stopped and other cost-saving opportunities. Ask your pharmacist to identify less expensive generic drugs, an available combination tablet that would be cheaper than getting two separate prescriptions, if there is one drug that might treat two health conditions, and of course, if any medications may no longer be needed.

Do not overlook the role of nondrug ways to manage your health conditions as a way to reduce costs. As discussed in Chapter 7, healthy lifestyle changes and other nondrug modifications can reduce the need for drug therapy. Another benefit is the possibility of fewer medications, which would help with adherence, too. Ask your physician to review with you the most effective nondrug strategies for managing your particular conditions and to update you about new recommendations.

Certain cost-saving suggestions that are widely touted should be approached with caution. Discount savings cards can look enticing and, in some situations, might be a good option. However, they do not work with insurance programs and will not count toward your deductible. Be careful about routinely shopping around at different pharmacies for better prices. The tradeoff is that you lose the ability of having a pharmacist know all that you are taking and to track drug interactions. In addition, you likely will not have the opportunity to get to know one pharmacist who can be your advocate when problems arise with your drug therapy. Finally, using free drug samples from your doctor's office might be a helpful short-term way to reduce costs; however, relying on samples long term can be risky. The supply at your physician's office might not be consistently available, leaving you in the lurch if samples run out. Furthermore, using drug samples means that the pharmacy will not have record of the medication, and safeguards such as drug interaction screening cannot occur.

Finally, be cautious about online pharmacies. There are many illegitimate pharmacies out there, and integrity of the product dispensed cannot be guaranteed. The National Association of Boards of Pharmacy accredits digital (online) pharmacies. Its website has a search function to find an accredited online pharmacy (see Resources section). The legality of importing medications from Canada has been addressed by presidential executive orders in recent years, but final rules are in flux and rest with individual states. Consumers are advised to check with current state and federal laws before opting for a Canadian pharmacy. Updates can be found at FDA.gov.

TALK ABOUT MEDICATION ADHERENCE

Adherence is hard, and we all need support at times. A family member or friend can help you stick with your drug therapy routine and remind you to take your medications. Ask your pharmacist to help make adherence easier for you. On request, the pharmacy can provide easy-open caps and possibly large-print material, for example. Ask your pharmacist for more information on the adherence aids mentioned earlier. If you feel overwhelmed or uncomfortable navigating any aspect of accessing your medications, managing them at home, or using the online resources, ask for assistance. Office staff and your clinicians want to support you. The internet can be intimidating if you do not know exactly what you are looking for. Your pharmacist, another trusted member of your health-care team, a family member, or a friend can guide you.

Most importantly, be honest with your health-care team about how you take your medications, especially if you sometimes intentionally are nonadherent. There are many reasons for nonadherence and no one is to blame. Together, you can address barriers, whether they result from bothersome side effects, high-cost, or doubt about the need for a medication. Clinicians cannot know your concerns if you do not share them. Your preferences and values matter.

SUMMARY

Taking medications on a routine basis can be challenging. Nonadherence is a major cause of medication-related problems and needs to be addressed in a collaborative manner. Ideally, patients and clinicians should work together to determine the best way to address each person's unique barriers. This chapter presented various tips and strategies that are useful for addressing the most common barriers that impact medication adherence in older adults. Pharmacists are an excellent resource to help individuals identify adherence barriers and navigate among the many options to address them. Individuals need to be proactive in managing their medications safely at home and ready to call on others for support when needed.

What You Can Do at Home

- Know what the correct instructions are for each medication.
- Get your medications refilled on time—don't wait until the last minute.
- Write up a schedule for when to take your medications; post it in a prominent place.

- Use a weekly pill organizer; keep it where you will see it every day to remind you.
- Use other reminder aids to help you remember to take your medications.
- Ask for support from a family member or friend when needed.

What You Can Do with Your Pharmacist

- Ask your pharmacist to simplify your medication schedule.
- Ask for a review of possible unnecessary drug therapy or drugs that indicate a prescribing cascade.
- Find out about different reminder aids to help with adherence and discuss which ones might be most effective for you.
- Ask about a medication synchronization program at your pharmacy to get your medications refilled on one day each month.
- Ensure you are using proper technique with your inhalers and eye drops; ask for instructions with new prescriptions and for a refresher at your annual medication review.
- Ask for ways to reduce costs, if cost of medications is a problem.
- If appropriate for your situation, ask about special packaging.

What You Can Do with Your Physician

- Be honest about how you take your medications at home and if you are skipping or forgetting doses.
- Speak up if you have trouble affording your medications; ask about ways to reduce costs, including nondrug therapy options.
- Make sure you are not taking unnecessary drug therapy or drugs that indicate a prescribing cascade, which can add medications and complicate your drug regimen.

RESOURCES

- Accredited Digital Pharmacies, by National Association of Boards of Pharmacy: https://nabp.pharmacy /programs/accreditations-inspections/digital-pharmacy /accredited-digital-pharmacies/
- BeSafeRx for online pharmacy information and tips: https://www.fda.gov/drugs /quick-tips-buying-medicines-over-internet /besaferx-your-source-online-pharmacy-information
- Must for Seniors: https://mustforseniors.org/
- Safe Pharmacy by the National Association of Boards of Pharmacy, information about online pharmacies: https://safe .pharmacy/
- Script your Future, tools to support adherence for selected disease states: https://scriptyourfuture.org /medication-adherence/
- Talk Before you Take, by BeMedWise: http://www .talkbeforeyoutake.org/

Chapter 18

Choose Nonprescription Products Carefully

Nonprescription products are widely used and offer the convenience of easy access and the ability to self-treat minor ailments. For the purposes of this book, I have taken the liberty of grouping together over-the-counter (OTC) medications and dietary supplements into the general bucket of nonprescription products. Recall from Chapter 6 that this is slightly unconventional; the separate categories of OTC drugs and dietary supplements are regulated in distinct ways by the Food and Drug Administration (FDA). While many of the recommendations can apply easily to either category, the specific issues are slightly different. Thus, most of the recommendations in this chapter are presented separately by category.

GENERAL CONSIDERATIONS

A few general considerations apply to both OTC products and dietary supplements. First of all, be mindful that both categories of nonprescription medications need to be viewed as medications. They have effects on the body, and the body works to metabolize (transform) and eliminate them as it does with any prescription drug. Thus, these products deserve the same kind of respect regarding adverse effects, interactions, and other medication-related problems.

Be sure to include all nonprescription products that you take on a regular basis on your medication list. Keeping a complete list helps to detect important interactions and adverse effects and avoid duplicated therapy. A story relayed by an ophthalmologist colleague illustrates the value of keeping a complete medication list and sharing it with your health-care professionals. Ray had glaucoma and began self-treatment of his allergies with an OTC steroid nasal spray, triamcinolone (Nasacort®). At his next eye exam, the eye doctor found Ray's eye pressure to be significantly increased. As it turned out, the nasal spray Ray started four months earlier was the source of the problem, which the doctor quickly identified. Ray stopped using that OTC product, which reversed this adverse drug reaction.

Another universal recommendation is to bring the actual bottles or packages of your nonprescription products to medical appointments and to every medication review. This avoids error or misunderstanding about what ingredients are in these products., An easier way for some to do this is to take a good photo of the label and ingredient information to show to your clinician. I always ask to see the original packaging when doing a medication review. "Calcium" can be calcium carbonate or calcium citrate, and the instructions for how to take each of these products is different. Clients have told me they take "Tylenol" (acetaminophen), when really it is Tylenol PM® that also contains diphenhydramine, a potentially inappropriate medication (PIM) for older adults (discussed in Chapter 10). Fish oil is another product notorious for being marketed with different amounts of the desired omega-3-fatty acids; thus, taking "1000 mg of fish oil" is meaningless without seeing the actual ingredients listed on the label.

TIPS FOR CHOOSING AND USING OTC PRODUCTS

Several recommendations are applicable mainly to OTC medications. Choose single-ingredient products when possible. This minimizes exposure to unnecessary medication and reduces the risk of interactions and adverse events. A multiple-ingredient product can be packaged to sound like it is the perfect solution for your ills. But it is more important to take only what you need. If your only symptom is nasal congestion, there is no need for a product that treats cough, pain, and fever, too.

Ask your pharmacist which OTC medicine is most effective for your situation. Do you need omeprazole or is famotidine or a liquid antacid the way to go? For congestion, should you choose a tablet or a nasal spray? Do you need a pain medicine that treats inflammation or will acetaminophen work? With so many options from which to choose, seeking advice on the best option to fit your needs can be invaluable.

Be aware that some of the OTC ingredients on the market are not well-suited for older adults. Namely, older antihistamines (so-called "first generation antihistamines") like diphenhydramine, chlorpheniramine, and doxylamine are identified by geriatrics experts as PIMs in older adults, as are nonsteroidal anti-inflammatory drugs (NSAIDs, such as ibuprofen and naproxen) when used long-term.[328] Note that OTC sleep products (like Tylenol PM® or Unisom®) all contain one of the older antihistamines because these agents cause sedation as a side effect. However, they are PIMs and should be avoided because they increase the risk of dry mouth, constipation, and confusion.

Avoid doubling or tripling up on an ingredient that is contained in more than one OTC product. This is another reason to avoid multiple-ingredient products and it reinforces the importance of knowing which active ingredients (medicines) are in the products you take. Acetaminophen is found in hundreds of products (OTC and prescription), which can lead to people ingesting more than they realize and developing liver damage because they exceeded the daily maximum. Cough and cold products contain various drug combinations that can lead to excessive and unrecognized ingestion of certain medications. Be aware of aspirin in OTC products, especially if you already take a daily aspirin for heart protection or another medication that increases bleeding risk (discussed in Chapter 11).

An eighty-year-old client I met with was experiencing decreased memory, increased tiredness, and recent falls. She was innocently taking a cough medicine that contained not only guaifenesin (to thin mucus in her lungs), but doxylamine, one of the older antihistamines mentioned that is potentially inappropriate for older individuals. She was taking it several times a day but did not include it on her list. I learned she was taking this product simply because it was sitting on her dining room table, and I asked her about it. Thus, her "cough medicine" was an important contributing factor to her drowsiness, fall risk, and quite possibly memory impairment.

Be alert to brand-name extensions, sound-alike drug names, or look-alike packaging (see Chapter 6). Read labels carefully or check with the pharmacist to make sure the ingredient you want is in the product you've chosen.

Find out about interactions with other drugs and health conditions. Interaction information is required on OTC labels, but may not be specific. For example, a health condition interaction might simply say "thyroid disease" or "heart disease." Do not overlook these warnings. If you are unsure if they apply to you, speak with the pharmacist.

Read the label to make sure you are taking the correct dose. Do not take it more often than stated and do not take more within a twenty-four-hour period than is recommended. Dangerous errors can occur when people do not pay attention to this information. Acetaminophen 650 mg is an extended-release formulation that should be dosed every eight hours, rather than the usual four- or six-hour interval with the regular preparation. Older adults can take ibuprofen every six hours, but naproxen only every twelve hours. When measuring liquid doses, household spoons are imprecise and should never be used. Instead, use an appropriate medication dosing cup. These usually are included with the product but can be purchased separately.

Don't take the product for longer than stated on the label. A common example where this error occurs is with proton pump inhibitors (PPIs, such as omeprazole), which should not be used for self-treatment of heartburn for more than two weeks.[329] Beyond two weeks of treatment, if symptoms persist, something more serious could be at play and medical evaluation is needed. Prolonged use also can lead to rebound acid production, which can make stopping a PPI difficult. This leads into the final recommendation for OTC products, which is to know when enough is enough. Any time you self-treat, it is important to know when to see a doctor if the condition does not improve. Examples here include self-treating stomach pain that could be an ulcer; or respiratory symptoms that could be bronchitis or pneumonia.

TIPS FOR CHOOSING AND USING DIETARY SUPPLEMENTS

Patients and consumers need to have a high level of skepticism when choosing a dietary supplement because of how they are regulated, as discussed in Chapter 6. The phrase "buyer beware" applies. Check with your pharmacist about safety and effectiveness before you spend money on a product. Many dietary supplements are of questionable benefit but are heavily marketed. Products that claim to boost memory or brain health, promote weight loss, or provide blood sugar support are examples of supplements that sound promising but lack clinical evidence. If a claim sounds too good to be true, it probably is.

Ask your pharmacist about possible interactions between the supplement and your prescription drugs and health conditions. For many products, there might not be much information available, while others have well-known interactions. Some of the supplements with known interactions include St. John's wort, calcium, and iron, for example. Several supplements are known to increase bleeding risk and can interact when taken with prescription medications that reduce the ability of the blood to clot—namely anticoagulants and antiplatelet agents, as well as aspirin (see Chapters 6 and 11).

Be cautious also about products that contain a proprietary blend of ingredients. These are multiple-ingredient products that have the potential to interact with your medications or health conditions. Because the individual ingredients often are not listed, or in some cases they may be quite numerous, it may not be feasible for the pharmacist to check for interactions or assess possible side effects.

Read the top of the Supplement Facts label to confirm the "serving size" for that product. This tells you the number of tablets or capsules that contain the stated amount on the front label. The label also provides general guidance on how many tablets or capsules to take, how many times per day, and if you should take the supplement with or without food. Remember that these dosing recommendations are provided by the supplement manufacturer and have not been approved by the FDA.

Finally, dietary supplements carry the risk of containing contaminants or being mislabeled. For example, a product might contain one or more ingredients that are not listed on the label. Conversely, there might be an ingredient that is stated on the label but not found in the actual product.[330] To have greater confidence in the quality of the supplement you purchase, choose a product that has a lot number and expiration date on the packaging. In addition, look for a seal of quality, such as "USP Verified" (by the United States Pharmacopeia), "NSF Certified" (by NSF International) or Consumer Labs (a private organization). These verifications indicate the product has been tested for quality and safety and that it contains what is stated on the label. More information is available on the websites of these agencies.

SUMMARY

OTC products and dietary supplements are available without a prescription. This means they are easily accessible; however, this also means that consumers can use these self-care products without insight or guidance from a health-care professional. Nonprescription products have the potential to contribute to adverse reactions, interactions, and other medication-related problems. For older individuals who take several medications and have multiple health conditions, choosing the right product is extremely important.

OTC products and dietary supplements need to be chosen carefully to minimize exposure to unnecessary, ineffective, and possibly harmful ingredients. Seeking the advice of your physician or pharmacist is an essential step to avoid medication-related problems and errors. This chapter provided tips and strategies to reduce the risk of problems and empower individuals to choose and use nonprescription products safely and effectively. No list can be 100 percent complete, but these recommendations offer a sound start.

What You Can Do at Home

- Include all OTC products and dietary supplements that you take on a regular basis on your medication list; keep it up to date.
- Read the instructions before taking the OTC product or dietary supplement; do not exceed the recommended amount in a twenty-four-hour period.

- For dietary supplements, read the label to note how many tablets make up a "serving size."
- Bring the actual products (bottles or packaging) or photos to your medication review or medical appointments.
- Don't take a product for longer than intended; check the information provided on the product label; seek medical help if symptoms do not improve or worsen.
- Use an approved medication dosing cup or syringe to measure the dose of a liquid medication; do not use a household spoon.
- Store medications in a cool, dry place, where they are safe from young children, grandchildren, and pets.
- Do not keep expired medications at home; clean out your medicine cabinet once a year (see Chapter 15 and **Box 15-2**).

What You Can Do with Your Pharmacist

- Share your *complete* medication list so the pharmacist can check for duplications, interactions, and adverse effects.
- Ask before buying a product. Is it effective? Is it safe for *your* situation? Is it necessary?
- Confirm that you are buying products only with the ingredients to treat your symptoms so as to avoid taking unnecessary medications.
- Confirm that the product you are buying does not interact with your health conditions; pay attention to the warning information on the OTC label.
- Check for drug interactions with the OTC product or dietary supplement.
- Get an annual medication review that includes your nonprescription medications.

What You Can Do with Your Physician

- Share your *complete* medication list with each of your physicians, especially before a new medication is added; be sure your list is up-to-date and includes all OTC products and dietary supplements you take on a regular basis.
- Discuss options for managing a new condition or symptom; ask about nonprescription options, as well as a "watch and wait" approach and other nondrug options that might be appropriate.
- Ask about appropriate duration for self-treating your symptoms; make an appointment to see your physician if symptoms are not improving as expected.

RESOURCES

- From the FDA:
  - Information for consumers on safe use of OTC products: https://www.fda.gov/about-fda/center-drug-evaluation -and-research-cder/consumer-information-safe-use-over -counter-drug-products
  - Information for consumers on using dietary supplements: https://www.fda.gov/food/dietary-supplements /information-consumers-using-dietary-supplements
  - Mixing medications and dietary supplements can endanger your health: https://www.fda.gov/consumers /consumer-updates/mixing-medications-and-dietary -supplements-can-endanger-your-health
  - FDA's Supplement Your Knowledge program (contains printable information and videos): https://www.fda.gov /food/information-consumers-using-dietary-supplements /supplement-your-knowledge

- Get Relief Responsibly, information about OTC pain medications: https://www.getreliefresponsibly.com/
- Acetaminophen Awareness Coalition, Know Your Dose: https://www.knowyourdose.org/

Chapter 19

Health and Drug Information on the Internet

The internet has become the go-to resource for just about everything, including health and drug information. Unfortunately, it is an unregulated world where we can find both good and bad material. Especially when it comes to health and drug information, material can be outdated, biased, or written by people without the proper qualifications. Naïve consumers can be duped into believing they are reading reliable information when in actuality it is a well-disguised advertisement. Thus, it is incredibly important to be mindful of your sources of health information when searching online. It is also important to verify the information you find with a clinician you trust, so that you are neither scared away from beneficial drug therapy nor swayed into trying an unproven treatment. Next is information that can help you evaluate the reliability of health- and drug-related websites.

Unless you have the proper training and background, it is safest not to rely solely on your own judgment to evaluate the information from an internet source. Seek confirmation and explanation from experts on your health-care team who can help you interpret the information as it applies to you.

GUIDELINES TO EVALUATE A HEALTH OR DRUG INFORMATION WEBSITE

The first consideration when looking at a website is to find out who is sponsoring or hosting it. Is it a nonprofit patient advocacy organization, the government, or a private company? If there are advertisements, how many and how prominently are they displayed? More reliable websites tend to end in ".gov," ".edu," or ".org." This is a general rule; there can be exceptions.

Who wrote the information on the website? Ideally there will be an author name and possibly also a reviewer. Is the author qualified to write on the topic? Health and drug information should be written by an appropriate health-care professional. Look for contact information for the author. If not listed with the author information, a credible website should have a tab such as "about us" or "contact us" that provides more information about who is responsible for the website, its purpose, and a way to reach someone. If the information is posted with no way to reach the author or the organization associated with the website, this can raise questions about the integrity of the information.

When was the article or information written? The date that the material originally was written and the date of when it was last reviewed or updated should be stated with the article. Medical and drug information can change rapidly. Depending on the topic, material can become outdated within a few years, if not sooner.

Consider the purpose of the website. Is it a patient advocacy organization that provides disease-specific information such as for Alzheimer's, Parkinson's, or heart disease? These tend to be more trustworthy. Or is it a commercial site that is selling a product? Some websites provide unbiased information, while others promote a personal opinion. Reputable websites will present a balance of information that is based on scientific evidence. Check for a reference list at the end of the article, for example, or links to studies embedded within the text. Be cautious about a webpage that makes unsupported claims or reports only on benefits without discussing side effects. If you are looking up information about a dietary supplement, for example, be careful about biases and underreporting of possible risks. Many of these sites are run by manufacturers who want you to buy their supplement. In other instances, a medical professional might have a website with information about dietary supplements but also sells a line of dietary supplements. Be careful to not be swayed too easily.

Because of the critical nature of health and drug information, it is wise to compare information from more than one credible website. There is much variability in the quality of health information on the internet. If the information is consistent between two or more reliable sources, you can feel more assured that the information can be trusted. If there are discrepancies, be sure to note them and seek clarification with your physician or pharmacist.

It is a fair assumption to say that at some point, we all have been or will be seekers of health and drug information on the internet. It is a reasonable place to start, but what matters is how we use that information. When a health-care decision is at stake, always discuss what you find on the internet with clinicians you trust.

SPECIFIC DRUG INFORMATION SOURCES

Drug information websites are a source of broad information about medications. They serve as a good starting place for individuals who want to review the essential information about their medications, for example. Common websites include Rxlist.com, Drugs.com, and Medlineplus.gov (see also **Box 19-1**). Generally, these websites have fairly reliable information. There are some drawbacks, too, to consider. Some of these websites provide so much information that it is hard to sift through it all and know what is most important. Others are simplified and may not provide enough information of value. Information specific to older adults may be limited or not included. Likewise, it might be difficult to know if certain drug interaction or dosage information applies to you. In addition, patients can be misled when they look up a medicine they were told is to treat their pain and find that it treats seizures, for example. Remember that some medications can be used for more than one reason, and sometimes a medication can be used for a condition other than what the FDA officially approved it to treat. This is referred to as "off-label" use, and drug information websites typically will not have information on off-label uses.

Many individuals turn to internet websites to check for drug interactions. A few cautionary words are in order about these drug interaction checker programs. Websites use different interaction databases, which means that you might find different results from different websites. It is easy to make an error when entering drug names, especially when individuals are not familiar with sound-alike or look-alike names, thus leading to incorrect results. In addition, not all programs include dietary supplements; however, most can screen for vitamin interactions. Some of the programs provide information on interactions with food, alcohol, and even cannabis (marijuana).

Probably the most important caution is that it can be difficult to interpret the drug interaction reports and what is meaningful to a particular individual. The significance of an interaction for you depends on route of administration of the medication, dosage, and other health information unique to you. Reports can look intimidating if many interactions are identified and have the potential to scare patients if a serious interaction is listed. As discussed earlier in this book, drug interactions are complex and need to be addressed on an individual basis. It is important that individuals do not make changes to their medications based solely on information found on the internet, be it from a drug information website or a drug interaction checker program. Always confirm what you find with health-care professionals you trust.

SELECTED HEALTH AND DRUG INFORMATION WEBSITES

Box 19-1 contains a listing of websites that have good reputations and offer reliable consumer information on various topics. However, information on these websites is not a substitute for medical advice from your health-care professionals. Always talk with your physician, pharmacist, or other members of your health-care team about the information you find to make sure it is accurate and applies to you.

If you are using the internet to augment your understanding of a health or medication situation, it is helpful to compare information from two or more sources to check for consistency. Never rely solely on the internet to make a health or medication decision. Use the information you find to open the conversation with your clinicians. Be mindful that drug information found on most websites will not address special considerations for older adults as described throughout this book. Websites with information specific to older adults also are noted in the listing in **Box 19-1**.

Box 19-1. Selected Health and Drug Information Websites and Related Resources

General health information:

- Health In Aging by the American Geriatrics Society (older adult specific): https://www.healthinaging.org/
- Mayo Clinic: https://www.mayoclinic.org /patient-care-and-health-information
- MedlinePlus, older adult health: https://medlineplus. gov/olderadulthealth.html
- MedlinePlus: https://medlineplus.gov/healthtopics.html
- My Health Finder (preventive health and wellness information): https://health.gov/myhealthfinder
- National Council on Aging: https://ncoa.org/older -adults, information for older adults on finances, health, and overall well-being
- National Institute on Aging, Health Information: https://www.nia.nih.gov/health
- National Institutes of Health, Health Information: https://www.nih.gov/health-information
- WebMD: https://www.webmd.com/

Drug information:

- Drugs.com: https://www.drugs.com/drug_information
  .html
- Medline Plus, Drugs, Herbs and Supplements:
  https://medlineplus.gov/druginformation.html
- WebMD: https://www.webmd.com/ (note that RxList.
  com is owned by WebMD)

Drug interaction checkers (always discuss this information with
your physician or pharmacist):

- Drugs.com: https://www.drugs.com/drug_interactions
  .html
- Medscape: https://reference.medscape.com
  /drug-interactionchecker
- RxList: https://www.rxlist.com/drug-interaction
  -checker.htm
- WebMD: https://www.webmd.com/interaction
  -checker/default.htm

Medication safety information:

- BeMedWise: https://www.bemedwise.org/
- Health In Aging by the American Geriatrics Society
  (older adult specific): https://www.healthinaging.org/
- Medication Safety Program, adverse drug events in
  adults, plus links to other resources: https://www.cdc
  .gov/medicationsafety/adult_adversedrugevents.html
- Resources for Consumers and Patients:
  https://www.fda.gov/drugs/resources-you-drugs
  /information-consumers-and-patients-drugs

- Safe Medication, by American Society of Health-system Pharmacists: https://www.safemedication.com/

Find a senior care pharmacist:

- HelpWithMyMeds.org, by the American Society of Consultant Pharmacists, national directory of senior care pharmacists: www.HelpWithMyMeds.org or https://www.ascp.com/mpage/Care_Pharmacist

Elder care locator:

- Nationwide service to connect older adults with local services, including Area Agencies on Aging: https://eldercare.acl.gov/Public/About/Index.aspx

SUMMARY

The internet contains a wealth of health- and drug-related information. Concerns are that the quality of information is highly variable. Plus, the information has the potential to be inaccurate, incomplete, or misleading. Inaccurate or misinterpreted information can lead to confusion, fear about drug therapy, or inappropriate self-treatment, all of which can cause serious harm. The internet will continue to grow as a resource of medical information for consumers. Individuals seeking health or drug information need to be savvy by using reliable websites and being cautious in how they interpret health and drug information on the internet. Information always should be discussed with a trusted health professional.

What You Can Do at Home

- Never rely solely on information from a website to make a decision about your medications or health.
- Do not stop or make changes to your medications based on something you read on the internet.
- Be mindful of the quality of the website when seeking health or drug information on the internet. Rely on trusted websites for health and drug information.
- Look for the author's name and date of when the material was written; take note of other clues as discussed in this chapter to evaluate the reliability of the website.

What You Can Do with Your Pharmacist

- Discuss drug information from the internet with your pharmacist to clarify and learn how the material applies to your situation.
- Ask about reliable websites the pharmacist trusts that can address your particular questions.
- Verify drug interaction and other drug information with your pharmacist. Never make changes to drug therapy on your own.

What You Can Do with Your Physician

- Discuss information from the internet with your physician to clarify and learn how the material applies to your situation.
- Ask about reliable websites the physician trusts that can address your particular questions.
- Verify drug and medical information with your physician. Never make changes to drug therapy on your own.

Afterword

Maybe It's Your Medications grew out of my experience, of course, but also out of my frustration with the status quo. My goal with this book is to set you up with greater awareness, knowledge, and plenty of tools to make a difference. I have explained why issues change regarding medication use as we get older and why this topic is important. I also have done my best to describe what you can do to reduce risks and improve the safety of medication use.

If you are ready to take an action to improve medication safety, but are not sure where to begin, a good first step is to find out more about the medications you take. Even if you already know quite a bit about your medications, there always is something more to learn or something you might have overlooked. Write out your complete medication list and start filling in the blanks. Ask your pharmacist or physician to take a few minutes to explain or review with you the reason for each medicine. Once you know the reasons, then you can dig further to the next level and ask about goals of treatment and what to look for, and so on. One question will lead to the next and ultimately to a valuable discussion about your health care.

It is clear we need to change the way we approach and view medications. We can do better as health-care professionals and as patients if we are able to support each other to improve medication use. I leave you with a few closing thoughts.

1. For patients, consumers, and family members: Don't go it alone with your health. This material is not a substitute for health-care professionals who know you. As I already have written many times, talk with your pharmacist or physician about your medications and the issues I have raised. The information in this book provides insight and guidance, not definitive answers. Take what

you learned here and interact with your physician, nurse, or pharmacist in a more meaningful way about your medications.

2. For health-care professionals: Be patient when patients come to you now with more questions about their drug therapy and asking for more information about non-drug strategies. If this book has done its job, this will become much more commonplace! The challenge is to keep the patient at the center of care while dealing with healthcare system protocols and expectations that compete for your attention.

3. For health-care systems and payers of health care: We need to place medication use in the bigger context of health care, wellness, and preventive care. Pharmacists need to be more accessible as part of the primary care team to improve medication use. Both prescribers and patients can benefit from a pharmacist's expertise as we all strive to optimize drug therapy. Nowhere is this more critical than in older individuals who too often experience the gaps in our health-care system.

As our population continues to age and health-care costs increase, there is no better time than the present to reassess our approach to medication use.

Glossary

Adherence (medication adherence): The extent to which an individual takes his or her medications according the instructions given by the prescriber; taking one's medications in the correct manner.

Adverse drug event: Any injury or harm caused by exposure to a medication. This is a broad term that includes adverse drug reactions, allergic reactions, and physical or mental harm.

Adverse drug reaction: Any unintended or harmful response to a medication when it is used for an accepted medical reason and at a usual and proper dose; a drug side effect.

Ageism: Stereotyping an individual based on age.

AGS Beers Criteria: A list of potentially inappropriate medications (PIMs) that should be used with caution or avoided *in certain situations* in adults age sixty-five and older. The criteria were developed by geriatrics experts as a resource to educate prescribers and consumers about medications for which the risk of possible harm is thought to outweigh clinical benefit. This highly respected list of PIMs is updated every three years by the American Geriatrics Society (AGS). (See potentially inappropriate medications)

Anticholinergic drugs: Medications that block cholinergic receptors in the nervous system and lead to a group of side effects that includes dry mouth, dry eyes, blurred vision, constipation, difficulty urinating, and confusion. Anticholinergic drugs or drugs with anticholinergic properties are particularly troublesome for older adults and should be avoided when possible.

Anticholinergic properties: Refers to side effects that result from anticholinergic medications (see anticholinergic drugs).

Anticoagulant drugs: Medications that block certain proteins in the blood that are involved in the body's system that regulates blood clot formation following injury to a blood vessel. These types of drugs are used clinically to reduce the ability to form a clot; thus, bleeding is a possible adverse drug reaction associated with anticoagulants.

Antihistamines, first generation: Medications that block histamine receptors; they commonly are used to treat allergies and allergic reactions. First generation refers to older antihistamines, which are associated with sedation and significant *anticholinergic effects*. Newer or second-generation antihistamines have little-to-no anticholinergic effects.

Antiplatelet drugs: Medications that reduce the ability of platelets to "stick" together to form a blood clot. Platelets are a component of the blood and part of the body's system that regulates clot formation following injury to a blood vessel. Antiplatelets are used clinically to reduce clot formation; thus, bleeding is a possible adverse drug reaction.

Antipsychotic drugs: Medications that are used to treat various psychiatric conditions such as schizophrenia and bipolar disorder; they sometimes are used off-label to manage difficult behaviors and psychological symptoms that occur in patients with dementia.

Appropriate polypharmacy: The judicious use of multiple medications, in which each medication has a valid clinical reason for use, is known to be effective, and does not cause significant side effects for the individual or the side effects are meaningfully outweighed by the benefits of the drug therapy. Appropriate polypharmacy needs to be distinguished from inappropriate polypharmacy (see also inappropriate polypharmacy, medication overload, and polypharmacy).

Beers Criteria (see AGS Beers Criteria)

Benzodiazepines: Class of medications that work by blocking specific receptors in the central nervous system causing it to slow down. These drugs commonly treat anxiety, insomnia, and/or seizures. Their side effects are particularly troublesome for older adults; thus, these drugs should be avoided when possible in this age group.

Beta blockers: Class of medications that work by blocking "beta receptors" throughout the body; beta blockers are used to treat high blood pressure, congestive heart failure, certain types of heart rhythm disturbances, among other heart-related conditions

Cardiovascular disease: Disease of the heart and blood vessels; some of the common cardiovascular diseases includes coronary artery disease, high blood pressure, heart attack, heart failure, peripheral artery disease, and stroke.

Central nervous system (CNS): The part of the body that includes the brain and spinal cord; it receives, processes, and responds to information from throughout the body. Medications that cross from the general blood circulation into the brain circulation are called centrally acting or CNS-active medications. Drugs that are CNS active can be associated with troublesome side effects in older adults such as drowsiness, dizziness, sedation, confusion, decreased memory, and fall risk.

Chronic: Long-term; a chronic condition is a health problem that lasts one year or longer and requires ongoing medical attention.

Decongestant: A medication that treats stuffy nose (nasal congestion); it can be taken orally (as tablets, capsules, or liquid formulations) or as a nasal spray. Decongestants are available without a prescription and commonly are included in cough and cold products.

Deprescribing: The process of reducing medication dosages or stopping medications that no longer are needed or no longer are of benefit to an individual. Deprescribing is part of the bigger approach of "right-sizing" or optimizing a person's medications to make sure the person is taking only the most appropriate doses and combination of medications.

Dietary supplements: Products intended to add or supplement the diet but are not conventional foods. Supplements generally are ingested (taken by mouth) and include plant-derived products (herbals and botanicals), vitamins, minerals, amino acids (proteins), and probiotics. They are regulated as food by the Food and Drug Administration.

Disease state: a health or medical condition; a specific diagnosis or illness.

Diuretics: Group of medications (a drug class) that commonly is used to treat high blood pressure and other cardiovascular conditions marked by water and salt (sodium) retention; commonly referred to as water pills. Diuretics work via the kidneys to increase the amount of water and sodium removed from the body and are associated with increased or more frequent urination.

Drug class: A group of medications that have the same mechanism of action (work in the same way). Examples of drug classes are beta blockers, proton pump inhibitors, and statin drugs. Medications within a drug class often (but not always) share similar side effects and are similarly effective.

Drug interaction: A reaction between two or more drugs that alters the effect of one or more of the drugs involved; drugs also can interact with health conditions (drug-disease interactions), as well as alcohol, food, and dietary supplements.

Drug regimen: The drug-therapy plan or schedule for a specific individual that describes when and how to take one's medications.

Endocrine system: A system in the body that is made up of several glands throughout the body that make different hormones; common disease states associated with the endocrine system are diabetes and diseases of the thyroid gland (hyper- or hypothyroidism).

Food and Drug Administration: The government agency that is responsible for overseeing the safety of the nation's food supply, medical products, medications, supplements, tobacco, cosmetics, and other public health-related areas.

Formulary: The preferred drug list for a specific hospital or insurance company. Medications that are "on formulary" are favored to be prescribed for patients based on effectiveness, safety, and/or cost considerations.

Health-care provider: A professional who is trained and licensed to deliver medical care or treatment, such as a physician, physician assistant, nurse, physical therapist, and pharmacist, among others. In some situations, a provider is more narrowly defined as a licensed professional who can bill for services.

Health-care team: Group of individuals that contributes to and coordinates the treatment and care of an individual; the team consists of various health-care professionals, family caregivers, and the individual who is receiving care; that is, the patient.

Hypertension: High blood pressure.

Hypoglycemia: Low blood sugar (glucose).

Inappropriate polypharmacy: Use of more medications than are clinically warranted; use of medications that are not clinically needed or that are harmful or not effective (see also appropriate polypharmacy, medication overload, and polypharmacy).

Indication (of a drug): The reason or purpose for a medication; knowing the indication of a medication allows the patient, pharmacist, and others on the health-care team to monitor and assess a drug's safety and effectiveness.

Medicare: The government health insurance coverage for adults age sixty-five and older, for some individuals younger than sixty-five with disabilities, and for people with end-stage kidney disease.

Medicare Part D: The prescription drug benefit for individuals enrolled in Medicare.

Medication adherence (see adherence)

Medication error: A mistake related to drug therapy that can occur at any point during the medication use process; medication errors are considered preventable events and have the potential to lead to medication related problems and patient harm (although most do not result in harm).

Medication overload: Use of multiple medications for which the risk of harm from a person's drug therapy is greater than the benefit (see also appropriate polypharmacy, inappropriate polypharmacy, and polypharmacy).

Medication reconciliation: The process of comparing the medications that are listed on a person's "official" medication list that is on record with one healthcare setting such as the hospital or a physician's office with what the person actually is taking at home; the process of identifying discrepancies between what the patient should be taking and what the patient actually is taking.

Medication regimen (see drug regimen)

Medication-related problem (MRP): An actual or potential event or issue associated with drug therapy that can interfere with a desired health outcome for an individual; eight types of medication-related problems have been identified that can help identify actual or potential problems during a medication review.

Medication use process: The stages that a medication "travels through" to reach the patient; stages include prescribing, transcribing or documenting the order, dispensing, administering, and monitoring.

Monitoring: The act of tracking or observing the effect of a medication on a patient over time, including both the desired effects and unwanted effects of drug therapy. Monitoring is one of the stages of the medication use process and a critical step to improving safe medication use.

Musculoskeletal system: The system in the body that is made up of bones, joints, muscles, tendons, and ligaments; common disease states associated with the musculoskeletal system are osteo- and rheumatoid arthritis, gout, muscle spasms, and low back pain.

Nonbenzodiazepines (nonBZDs): Class of medications that work by blocking specific receptors in the central nervous system causing it to slow down. These drugs are sedative-hypnotic agents that treat insomnia. Their side effects are particularly troublesome for older adults; thus, these drugs should be avoided when possible in this age group.

Nonprescription: Medications that can be obtained by the consumer or patient without needing a written order or prescription from a health-care provider.

NSAIDs (non-steroidal anti-inflammatory drugs): Medications that treat pain and inflammation; some NSAIDs require a prescription, while others are available without a prescription.

Off-label use: Use of a medication for a condition other than what the Food and Drug Administration approved the drug to treat.

Over-the-counter (OTC) products: Medications that can be accessed by patients and consumers without a prescription; they are regulated as drugs by the Food and Drug Administration; "OTC" and "nonprescription" often are used interchangeably.

Patient engagement: The desire and ability of individuals to be actively involved in their health choices and management with the goal of improving health outcomes and one's health-care experience.

Person-centered care (patient-centered care): Care that focuses on individual preferences and what matters most to an individual regarding his or her health-care decisions; patient-centered care. Person-centered care is a key component of shared-decision making.

Pharmaceutical: Relating to the preparation, manufacturing, sale, or use of medicinal drugs.

Pharmacodynamics: The science of the body's response to a drug, or, in other words, how the drug affects the body.

Pharmacokinetics: The science of how the body handles a drug once it is introduced into the body; what the body does to the drug to ultimately process it and get rid of it from the body. Pharmacokinetics consists of four stages: absorption, distribution, metabolism, and elimination.

Polypharmacy: The use of multiple medications, commonly defined as five or more; more precisely, it can be divided into appropriate and inappropriate polypharmacy (see also appropriate polypharmacy, inappropriate polypharmacy, and medication overload).

Potential prescribing omission: The absence of a medication that potentially could be beneficial for an older adult to treat or prevent a health condition; under-prescribing.

Potentially inappropriate medications (PIMs): Medications for which the potential for an unwanted or adverse effect is thought to be greater than the clinical benefits in adults age sixty-five and older, especially when there are safer or more effective choices available. (See AGS Beers Criteria and STOPP)

Prescriber: A healthcare professional who has legal authority to prescribe medications for an individual.

Prescribing inertia: The tendency for a prescriber to renew and continue prescription medications even though they may no longer be needed or appropriate for the patient.

Proton pump inhibitors (PPIs): Class of medications that inhibit acid production in the stomach; PPIs are used to prevent and treat stomach ulcers and gastroesophageal reflux disease.

Provider: (see healthcare provider)

Sedative-hypnotics: Medications that cause sedation and are used to treat insomnia such as benzodiazepines and nonbenzodiazepines; they have a slowing or calming effect in the brain (central nervous system). Sedative-hypnotic agents are associated with important side effects in older adults.

Shared decision making: A process in which patients (and family members) are fully informed about treatment options and participate with their clinicians to make healthcare decisions. The process ideally takes into account patient preferences and health goals plus the healthcare professional's knowledge and experience.

START criteria: A list of medications that are considered to be of particular value to older adults in preventing or treating certain health conditions; absence or omission of these medications is considered to be potentially inappropriate, depending on the patient's situation. START stands for Screening Tool to Alert to Right Treatment and is the companion document to the STOPP criteria.

STOPP criteria: A list of potentially inappropriate medications (PIMs) that are recommended to be avoided in adults age sixty-five and older in certain situations because the potential risks (adverse events) are considered to be greater than benefit. STOPP stands for Screening Tool of Older People's Prescriptions and is the companion document to the START criteria. (See potentially inappropriate medications)

Therapeutic: Tending to improve health; beneficial to one's health.

Acknowledgments

Thanks to my agent Eric Myers of Myers Literary Management, LLC, for recognizing the need and believing this book is important enough.

Thanks to my Skyhorse editor Caroline Russomanno for believing in the book, for your generous understanding when life gave me a few hiccups, and for your amazing editing skills.

Thanks to my friends, family, and colleagues who supported me throughout, even before this book came to be. To Ann R. Bannes, Brett Barenholtz, and Debra K. Schuster for your help at the very early stages. To Christine Antis, Devorah Barenholtz, Anika Hannah, Virginia Renz Higgins, Deroda McGrath, Suzanne Sierra Sewell, and Michele Wicks for being my readers and critics at the final stages. You all were there when I needed you to read and review, and you propped me up when I doubted it all. Special shout out to my writing buddies Virginia and Michele; your presence has been a blessing.

Thanks to my pharmacist colleagues for your professional viewpoints. You were indispensable with your comments and suggestions: Rhonda L. Bilger, Cindy Doran, Randy C. Hatton, Marsha Meyer, and William "Si" Simonson. To Marsha and Si, thank you for sharing my passion for senior care pharmacy; your perspectives and reassurance were instrumental.

Thanks to my brother Brett, we shared this journey for decades and you encouraged me that this book needs to be written. To my sister Devorah for helping me whenever I asked, from the earliest versions to the final manuscript. Thanks to Connie for your quiet reassurance and inspiration. To my mom and dad, whom I know are so proud of this final product.

Finally, thanks to Don, my partner through every up and down. You refused to let my self-doubt win out. Your viewpoint as a physician was invaluable. Thanks for reviewing every chapter and saving me when I got stuck finding the right words. Mostly, thanks for a few good belly laughs along the way.

Notes

Chapter 1

1 Megan Jaynes and Avinash B. Kumar, "The risks of long-term use of proton pump inhibitors: a critical review," *Therapeutic Advances in Drug Safety*, vol. 10 2042098618809927. (November 19, 2018). doi:10.1177/2042098618809927.

2 A profile of older Americans: 2021, Administration on Aging, Administration for Community Living, US Department of Health and Human Services (November 2022) https://acl.gov/aging-and-disability-in-america/data-and-research/profile -older-americans (accessed 2/12/23).

3 Kaiser Family Foundation, "A short look at long-term care for seniors," *Journal of the American Medical Association* 310, no.8 (2013):786.

4 A profile of older Americans: 2021.

5 Center for Disease Control and Prevention, Therapeutic Drug Use. Health, United States, 2019, table 39 (accessed September 1, 2022), https://www.cdc.gov/nchs /fastats/drug-use-therapeutic.htm.

6 Centers for Medicare and Medicaid Services, Chronic conditions among Medicare beneficiaries, Chartbook 2012 Edition. Baltimore, MD 2012.

7 David Lassman, Micah Hartman, Benjamin Washington, Kimberly Andrews, and Aaron Catlin, "US health spending trends by age and gender: selected years 2002-10," *Health Affairs* 33, no.5 (May 2014):815-22.

8 NHE fact sheet (National Health Expenditure Data), (https://www.cms.gov/research -statistics-data-and-systems/statistics-trends-and-reports/nationalhealthexpenddata /nhe-fact-sheet.html (accessed 3/10/19).

9 Lassman et al., "US health spending trends by age and gender: selected years 2002-10."

10 Nadine Shehab, Maribeth C. Lovegrove, Andrew I. Geller, Kathleen O. Rose, Nina J. Weidle, and Daniel S. Budnitz, "US emergency department visits for outpatient adverse drug events, 2013-2014," *Journal of the American Medical Association* 316, no.20 (November 22/29, 2016):2115-25.

11 Ibid.

12 CDC. Chronic diseases in America, https://www.cdc.gov/chronicdisease/resources /infographic/chronic-diseases.htm, Updated 1/12/21 (accessed 1/15/21).

13 Jonathan H. Watanabe, Terry McInnis, and Jan D. Hirsch, "Cost of prescription drug-related morbidity and mortality," *Annals of Pharmacotherapy* 52, no.9 (September 2018):829-37.

14 Deaths and Mortality, Center for Disease Control and Prevention, National Center for Health Statistics, https://www.cdc.gov/nchs/fastats/deaths.htm (accessed 1/15/21)

15 Alex Z. Fu, Jenny Z. Jiang, Jaxk H. Reeves, Jack E. Fincham, Gordon G. Liu, and Matthew Perri, "Potentially inappropriate medication use and healthcare expenditures in the US community-dwelling elderly," *Medical Care* 45, no.5 (May 2007):472-6.

16 10 Essential facts about Medicare and prescription drug spending, Kaiser Family Foundation, January 29, 2019, https://www.kff.org/infographic/10-essential-facts -about-medicare-and-prescription-drug-spending/ (accessed 3/10/19).

17 Sarah E. Brotherton and Sylvia I. Etzel, "Graduate medical education, 2019-2020," *Journal of the American Medical Association* 328, no. 11 (September 20, 2022):1230-50.

18 Kathryn E. Callahan, Nina Tumosa, and Rosanne M. Leipzig. "Big 'G' and little 'g' geriatrics education for physicians," *Journal of the American Geriatrics Society* 65, no. 10 (October 2017):2313-2317.

19 Geriatric Pharmacist Fact Sheet, www.BPSweb.org (accessed 1/28/18).

20 Bureau of Labor and Statistics, www.bls.gov/oes (accessed 1/28/18).

21 Anon. What is Gerontology? Geriatrics? Gerontology Society of America, n.d. [online]. Available at https://www.geron.org/images/gsa/AGHE/AGHEgerontologyandgeriatrics .pdf (accessed 2/1/23).

22 Donald M. Berwick, Thomas W. Nolan, and John Whittington. "The triple aim: care, health, and cost," *Health Affairs* 27, no.3 (May-June 2008):759-769. doi: 10.1377/hlthaff.27.3.759.

23 Choosing Wisely, https://www.choosingwisely.org/.

24 Katie Coleman, Edward Wagner, Judith Schaefer, Robert Reid, and Lisa LeRoy, "Redefining Primary Care for the 21st Century," White Paper (Prepared by Abt Associates, in partnership with the MacColl Center for Health Care Innovation and Bailit Health Purchasing, Cambridge, MA, under Contract No.290-2010-00004-I/290-32009-T). AHRQ Publication No. 16(17)-0022-EF. Rockville, MD: Agency for Healthcare Research and Quality; October 2016.

25 Judith Garber and Shannon Brownlee, "Medication overload: America's other drug problem," Brookline, MA: The Lown Institute, (2019) https://lowninstitute.org/projects /medication-overload-how-the-drive-to-prescribe-is-harming-older-americans/.

26 Working Group on Medication Overload, Eliminating medication overload: a national action plan, Brookline, MA: The Lown Institute, (2020) https://lowninstitute.org /reports/eliminating-medication-overload-a-national-action-plan/.

27 Anon, What is gerontology? Geriatrics?

28 Frank Molnar and Christopher C. Frank, "Optimizing geriatric care with the Geriatric 5Ms," *Canadian Family Physician* 65, no.1 (January 2019):39.

29 Choosing Wisely.

30 Coleman, "Redefining Primary Care for the 21st Century."

31 Garber, "Medication overload: America's other drug problem."

32 Working Group on Medication Overload, Eliminating medication overload: a national action plan.

Chapter 2

33 A profile of older Americans: 2021, Administration on Aging, Administration for Community Living, US Department of Health and Human Services (November 2022)   https://acl.gov/aging-and-disability-in-america/data-and-research/profile -older-americans (accessed 2/12/23).

34 David Lassman, Micah Hartman, Benjamin Washington, Kimberly Andrews, and Aaron Catlin, "US health spending trends by age and gender: selected years 2002- 10," *Health Affairs* 33, no.5 (May 2014): 815-22.

35 Center for Disease Control and Prevention, Therapeutic Drug Use. Health, United States, 2019, table 39 (accessed September 1, 2022), https://www.cdc.gov/nchs /fastats/drug-use-therapeutic.htm.

36 Ibid.

37 Ira B. Wilson, Cathy Schoen, Patricia Neuman, Michelle K. Strollo, William H. Rogers, Hong Chang, and Dana G. Safran, "Physician-patient communication about prescription medication nonadherence: a 50-state study of America's seniors," *Journal of General Internal Medicine* 22, no. 1 (January 2007): 6-12. DOI; 10.1007/ sll606-006-0093-0.

38 Jacqueline L. Green, Jonathan N. Hawley, and Kimberly J. Rask, "Is the number of prescribing physicians an independent risk factor for adverse drug events in an elderly outpatient population?" *American Journal of Geriatric Pharmacotherapy* 5, no.1 (March 2007): 31-39.

39 Niteesh K. Choudhry, Michael A. Fischer, Jerry Avorn, Josua N. Liberman, Sebastian Schneeweiss, Juliana Pakes, Troyen A. Brennan, and William H. Shrank, "The implications of therapeutic complexity on adherence to cardiovascular medications," *Archives of Internal Medicine* 171, no. 9 (May 9, 2011): 814-22.

40 Michael L. Barnett, Asaf Bitton, Jeff Souza, and Bruce E. Landon, "Trends in outpatient care for Medicare beneficiaries and implications for primary care, 2000 to 2019," *Annals of Internal Medicine* 174, no. 12 (December 2021): 1658-1665. doi:10.7326/M21-1523.

41 Green et al., "Is the number of prescribing physicians an independent risk factor for adverse drug events in an elderly outpatient population?"

42   Emily R. Hajjar, Joseph T. Hanlon, Richard J. Sloane, Catherine I. Lindblad, Carl F. Pieper, Christine M. Ruby, Laurence C. Branch, and Kenneth E. Schmader, "Unnecessary drug use in frail older people at hospital discharge," *Journal of the American Geriatrics Society* 53, no. 9 (September 2005): 1518-1523.

43   Choudry et al., "The implications of therapeutic complexity on adherence to cardiovascular medications."

44   Richard A. Hansen, Corrine I. Voils, Joel F. Farley, Benjamin J. Powers, Linda L. Sanders, Betsy Sleath, and Matthew L. Maciejewski, "Prescriber continuity and medication adherence for complex patients," *Annals of Pharmacotherapy* 49, no. 3 (March 2015): 293-302.

45   Green et al., "Is the number of prescribing physicians an independent risk factor for adverse drug events in an elderly outpatient population?"

46   Krista L. Donohoe, Elvin T. Price, Tracey L. Gendron, and Patricia W. Slattum, "Geriatrics: the aging process in humans and its effects on physiology," Chapter e22. In: JT Dipiro, GC Yee, M Posey, ST Haines, TD Nolin, and V Ellingrod, eds. *Pharmacotherapy a Pathophysiologic Approach*, 11th ed. New York, NY: McGraw-Hill Education; 2019, https://accesspharmacy-mhmedical-com.stlcopisa.uhsp.edu/book.aspx?bookid=2577#219306043 (Accessed December 1, 2021).

47   A. Clara Drenth-van Maanen, Ingeborg Wilting, and Paul A.F. Jansen, "Prescribing medicines to older people—how to consider the impact of ageing on human organ and body functions," *British Journal of Clinical Pharmacology* 86, no. 10 (October 2020): 1921-1930.

48   Anders Helldén, Ulf Bergman, Mia von Euler, Maria Hentschke, Ingegerd Oda-Cederlöf, and Gunner Öhlen, "Adverse drug reactions and impaired renal function in elderly patients admitted to the emergency department," *Drugs and Aging* 26, no.7 (2009): 595-606.

49   Mark W. Bowie and Patricia W. Slattum, "Pharmacodynamics in older adults: a review," *American Journal of Geriatric Pharmacotherapy* 5, no. 3 (September 2007): 263-303.

50   Donohoe, "Geriatrics: the aging process in humans and its effects on physiology."

51   Flora Chang, Ann M. O'Hare, Yinghui Miao, and Michael A. Steinman, "Use of renally inappropriate medications in older veterans: a national study," *Journal of the American Geriatrics Society* 63, no. 11 (November 2015): 2290-2297.

52   Donohoe, "Geriatrics: the aging process in humans and its effects on physiology."

53   Chang et al., "Use of renally inappropriate medications in older veterans: a national study."

54   Jesse A. Berlin, Susan C. Glasser, and Susan S. Ellenberg, "Adverse event detection in drug development: recommendations and obligations beyond phase 3," *American Journal of Public Health* 98, no. 8 (August 2008): 1366-71.

55 Stephen A. Goldman, Dianne L. Kennedy, and Ronald Lieberman, "Clinical therapeutics and the recognition of drug-induced disease," *MedWatch Continuing Education Article*, June 1995, Center for Drug Evaluation and Research, Food and Drug Administration.

56 Januvia Product Information, Merck & Co, Inc., 2021, Whitehouse Station, NJ (Accessed April 2, 2022).

57 Motegrity Product Information, Takeda, 2020, Lexington, MA (Accessed April 2, 2022).

58 Karen E. Lasser, Paul D. Allen, Steffie J. Woolhandler, David U. Himmelstein Sidney M. Wolfe, and David H. Bor, "Timing of new black box warnings and withdrawals for prescription medications," *Journal of the American Medical Association* 287, no. 17 (May 1, 2002): 2215-2220.

59 Schiff et al., "Principles of conservative prescribing."

Chapter 3

60 Patricia W. Slattum and Janice B. Schwartz. "A challenge: the American Geriatrics Society needs to address the lack of inclusion of older adults in new drug evaluation," (commentary) *Journal of the American Geriatrics Society* 69, no. 9 (September 2021): 2684-2688.

61 International Conference on Harmonisation of Technical Requirements for Registration of Pharmaceuticals for Human Use, Guidance for Industry, E7 studies in support of special populations: geriatrics, questions and answers, US Department of Health and Human Services, February 2012.

62 National Institutes of Health, NIH Grants and Funding online. Inclusion across the lifespan, Updated February 9, 2022 (Accessed March 30, 2022),https://grants.nih .gov/policy/inclusion/lifespan.htm.

63 Catherine Y. Spong and Diana W. Bianchi, "Improving public health requires inclusion of underrepresented populations in research" (Viewpoint) *Journal of the American Medical Association* 319, no. 4 (January 23, 2018): 337-338.

64 Trevor Hinshaw, Joan Kapusnik-Uner, Barbara Zarowitz, and Karl Matuszewski, "Identifying knowledge gaps in the labeling of medications for geriatric patients," *P&T* 38, no. 9 (September 2013): 535, 537-40.

65 Donna M. Lisi, "Specific prescribing information for geriatric use in the 2019 product labeling for novel new drug approvals," *Senior Care Pharmacist* 36, no. 9 (September 2021): 455-465.

66 Gordon D. Schiff, William L. Galanter, Jay Duhig, Amy E. Lodolce, Michael J. Koronkowski, and Bruce L. Lambert, "Principles of conservative prescribing," *Journal of the American Medical Association* 171, no. 16 (September 12, 2011): 1433-1440.

67 Helen W. Sullivan, Kathyrn J.Aikin, Kathleen T. David, Jennifer Berktold, Karen L. Stein, and Victoria J. Hoverman, "Consumer understanding of the scope of the FDA's prescription drug regulatory oversight: a nationally representative survey," *Pharmacoepidemiology and Drug Safety* 29, no.2 (February 2020): 134-40. doi: 10.1002/pds.4914.

68 Charles D. Hepler and Linda M. Strand, "Opportunities and responsibilities in pharmaceutical care," *American Journal of Hospital Pharmacy* 47, no.3 (March 1990): 533-543.

69 Hepler and Strand, "Opportunities and responsibilities in pharmaceutical care."

70 Jonathan H. Watanabe, Jerry McInnis, and Jan D. Hirsch, "Cost of prescription drug-related morbidity and mortality," *Annals of Pharmacotherapy* 52, no.9 (September 2018): 829-837. doi: 10.1177/1060028018765159.

71 Daniel S. Budnitz, Nadine Shehab, Maribeth C. Lovegrove, Andrew I. Geller, Jennifer N. Lind, and Daniel A. Pollock, "US emergency department visits attributed to medication harms, 2017-2019." *Journal of the American Medical Association* 326, no.13 (October 5, 2021): 1299-1309. doi: 10.1001/jama.2021.13844.

72 Nadine Shehab, Maribeth C. Lovegrove, Andrew I. Geller, Kathleen O. Rose, Nina J. Weidle, and Daniel S. Budnitz, "US emergency department visits for outpatient adverse drug events, 2013-2014," *Journal of the American Medical Association* 316, no.20 (November 22/29, 2016): 2115-25. doi: 10.1001/jama.2016.16201.

73 Jerry H. Gurwitz, Terry S. Field, Leslie R. Harrold, Jeffrey Rothschild, Kristin Debellis, Andrew C. Seger, et al., "Incidence and preventability of adverse drug events among older persons in the ambulatory setting," *Journal of the American Medical Association* 289, no. 9 (March 5, 2003): 1107-1116. doi: 10.1001/jama.289.9.1107.

74 Munir Pirmohamed, Sally James, Shaun Meakin, Chris Green, Andrew K. Scott, Thomas J. Walley, et al., "Adverse drug reactions as cause of admission to hospital: prospective analysis of 18 820 patients," *British Medical Journal* 329, no. 7456 (July 3, 2004): 15-19. doi: 10.1136/bmj.329.7456.15.

75 Khokan C. Sikdar, Reza Alaghehbandan, Don Macdonald, Brendan Barrett, Kayla D. Collins, Jennifer Donnan, et al. "Adverse drug events in adult patients leading to emergency department visits," *Annals of Pharmacotherapy* 44, no.4 (April 2010): 641-649. DOI 10.1345/aph.1M416.

76 Leslie Jo Samoy, Peter J. Zed, Kerry Wilbur, Robert M. Balen, Riyad B. Abu-Laban, and Mark Roberts, "Drug-related hospitalizations in a tertiary care internal medicine service of a Canadian hospital: a prospective study," *Pharmacotherapy* 26, no.11 (November 2006): 1578-86. doi: 10.1592/phco.26.11.1578

77 Gurwitz et al., "Incidence and preventability of adverse drug events among older persons in the ambulatory setting."

78 Daniel S. Budnitz, Daniel A. Pollock, Kelly N. Weidenbach, Aaron B. Mendelsohn, Thomas J. Schroeder, and Joseph L. Annest, "National surveillance of emergency department visits for outpatient adverse drug events," *Journal of the American Medical Association* 296, no.15 (Ocotober 18, 2006): 1858-1866.

79 Samoy et al., "Drug-related hospitalizations in a tertiary care internal medicine service of a Canadian hospital: a prospective study."

80 Carole P. Kaufman, Dominik Stämpfli, Kurt E. Hersberger, and Markus L. Lampert, "Determination of risk factors for drug-related problems: a multidisciplinary triangulation process," *BMJ Open* 5, no.3 (March 20, 2015): e006376. doi:10.1136/ bmjopen-2014-006376.

81 Heini Kari, Hanna Kortejärvi, Marja Airaksinen, and Raisa Laaksonen, "Patient involvement is essential in identifying drug-related problems," *British Journal of Clinical Pharmacology* 84, no.9 (September 2018): 2048-2058. doi: 10.1111/ bcp.13640.

82 Hedva B. Levy, "Self-administered medication risk questionnaire in an elderly population," *Annals of Pharmacotherapy* 37, no.7-8 (July-August 2003): 982-987. doi: 10.1345/aph.1C305.

83 Emmi Puumalainen, Marja Airaksinen, Sanni E. Jalava, Timothy F. Chen, and Maarit Dimitrow, "Comparison of drug-related problem risk assessment tools for older adults: a systematic review," *European Journal of Clinical Pharmacology* 76, no.3 (March 2020): 337-348. doi: 10.1007/s00228-019-02796-w.

84 Cori Gray, Catherine E. Cooke, and Nichole Brandt, "Evolution of Medicare Part D medication management program from inception in 2006 to present," *American Health and Drug Benefits* 12, no.5 (September 2019): 243-251.

85 Medication Therapy Management. Center for Medicare and Medicaid Services, Last modified 2/22/22 (Accessed April 16, 2022), https://www.cms.gov/Medicare/Prescription -Drug-Coverage/PrescriptionDrugCovContra/MTM#:~:text=Requirements%20 for%20Medication%20Therapy%20Management,the%20risk%20of%20adverse%20 events.

86 Antoinette B. Coe, Julie P.W. Bynum, and Karen B. Farris, "Comprehensive Medication Review: New Poll Indicates Interest but Low Receipt Among Older Adults," *JAMA Health Forum* 1, no. 10 (October 9, 2020): e201243. doi: 10.1001/ jamahealthforum.2020.1243.

Chapter 4

87 NeedyMeds BeMedWise Patient Information and Education, "Talk About Your Medicines Month Archive: 2016: Polypharmacy—America's Other Drug Problem," (Accessed April 25, 2022) https://www.bemedwise.org/talk-about-your-medicines -month-2019/

88   Teresa Carr, "Too Many Meds?" *Consumer Reports*, September 2017.

89   Judith Garber and Shannon Brownlee, "Medication overload: America's other drug problem," Brookline, MA: The Lown Institute, 2019, https://lowninstitute .org/projects/medication-overload-how-the-drive-to-prescribe-is-harming-older -americans/

90   Working Group on Medication Overload, "Eliminating medication overload: a national action plan," Brookline, MA: The Lown Institute, 2020.

91   Get the Medications Right Institute, About Us (Accessed April 25, 2022), https://gtmr.org/about/.

92   Lisa Esposito, "When Less May Be More: Many older patients could benefit from 'deprescribing,'" *U.S. News and World Report*, Best Hospitals 2021 edition.

93   Nashwa Masnoon, Sepehr Shakib, Lisa Kalisch-Ellett, and Gillian E. Caughey, "What is polypharmacy? A systematic review of definitions," *BMC Geriatrics* 17, no. 1, article no. 230 (October 10, 2017), doi:10.1186/s12877-017-0621-2.

94   Health, United States, 2019—Data Finder. National Center for Health Statistics, (Accessed May 22, 2022), https://www.cdc.gov/nchs/hus/contents2019 .htm#Table-039.

95   Masnoon et al., "What is Polypharmacy? A Systematic Review of Definitions."

96   Najwa Taghy, Linda Cambon, Jean-Marie Cohen, and Claude Dussart, "Failure to reach a consensus in polypharmacy definition: an obstacle to measuring risks and impacts—results of a literature review," *Therapeutics and Clinical Risk Management* 16 (February 2020): 57-73.

97   Garber, "Medication overload: America's other drug problem," p. 4.

98   Ibid.

99   Working Group on Medication Overload, "Eliminating medication overload: a national action plan."

100   Ibid.

101   Ibid, p. 72.

102   Centers for Medicare and Medicaid Services, Chronic conditions, chartbook and charts, Chronic condition charts: 2018, (Accessed April 26, 2022), https://www .cms.gov/Research-Statistics-Data-and-Systems/Statistics-Trends-and-Reports /Chronic-Conditions/Chartbook_Charts.

103   Peter Boersma, Lindsey I. Black, and Brian W. Ward, "Prevalence of multiple chronic conditions among US adults, 2018," *Preventing Chronic Disease* 17 (September 17, 2020): E106. doi:10.5888/pcd17.200130.

104   New drugs at FDA: CDER's new molecular entities and new therapeutic biological products, (Accessed April 26, 2022), https://www.fda.gov/drugs/development -approval-process-drugs/new-drugs-fda-cders-new-molecular-entities-and-new -therapeutic-biological-products.

105 United States Government Accountability Office, "Medicare spending on drugs with direct-to-consumer advertising," (May 18, 2021): GAO-21-380.

106 Richard G. Stefanacci, "Too much good can be bad," (editorial), *Assisted Living Consult* (March/April 2009): 8, 9, 11.

107 Terri R. Fried, Mary E. Tinetti, and Lynne Iannone, "Primary care clinicians' experiences with treatment decision making for older persons with multiple conditions," *Archives of Internal Medicine* 171, no.1 (January 10 2011): 75-80.

108 Cynthia M. Boyd, Jonathan Darer, Chad Boult, Linda P. Fried, Lisa Boult, and Albert W. Wu, "Clinical practice guidelines and quality of care for older patients with multiple comorbid diseases," *Journal of the American Medical Association* 294, no. 6 (August 10, 2005): 716-24.

109 Stefanacci, "Too much good can be bad."

110 Wesley Yin, Anirban Basu, James X. Zhang, Atonu Rabbani, David O. Meltzer, and G. Caleb Alexander, "The effect of the Medicare Part D prescription benefit on drug utilization and expenditures," *Annals of Internal Medicine* 148, no.3 (February 5, 2008): 169-77.

111 Anne D. Halli-Tierney, Catherine Scarbrough, and Dana Carroll, "Polypharmacy: evaluating risks and deprescribing," *American Family Physician* 100, no.1 (July 1, 2019): 32-8.

112 Emily Reeve, Lee-Fay Low, and Sarah N. Hilmer, "Attitudes of older adults and caregivers in Australia toward deprescribing," *Journal of the American Geriatrics Society* 67, no.6 (June 2019): 1204-10.

113 Emily Reeve, Jennifer L. Wolff, Maureen Skehan, Elizabeth A. Bayliss, Sarah N. Hilmer, and Cynthia M. Boyd, "Assessment of attitudes toward deprescribing in older Medicare beneficiaries in the United States," *JAMA Internal Medicine* 178, no.12 (December 1, 2018): 1673-1680.

114 Denise L. Arnoldussen, Karen Keijsers, Judith Drinkwaard, Wilma Knol, and Rob J. van Marum, "Older patients' perceptions of medicines and willingness to deprescribe," *Senior Care Pharmacist* 36, no.9 (September 2021): 444-454.

115 Holly M. Holmes and Adam Todd, "The role of patient preferences in deprescribing," *Clinics in Geriatric Medicine* 33, no.2 (May 2017): 165-175.

116 Paula A. Rochon, Mirko Petrovic, Antonio Cherubini, Graziano Onder, Denis O'Mahony, Shelley A. Sternberg, Nathan M. Stall, and Jerry H. Gurwitz, "Polypharmacy, inappropriate prescribing, and deprescribing in older people: through a sex and gender lens," *Lancet, Healthy Longevity* 2, no.5 (May 2021): e290-300.

117 Ibid.

118 Holmes et al., "The role of patient preferences in deprescribing," 165-175.

Chapter 5

119 Amanda Lavan and Paul Gallagher, "Predicting risk of adverse drug reactions in older adults," *Therapeutic Advances in Drug Safety* 7, no. 1 (2016): 11-22.

120 Nadine Shehab, Maribeth C. Lovegrove, Andrew I. Geller, Kathleen O. Rose, Nina J. Weidle, and Daniel S. Budnitz, "US emergency department visits for outpatient adverse drug events, 2013-2014," *Journal of the American Medical Association* 316, no. 20 (November 22/29, 2016): 2115-25.

121 Scott M. Vouri, Joseph S. van Tuyl, Margaret A. Olsen, Hong Xian, and Mario Schootman, "An evaluation of a potential calcium channel blocker—lower-extremity edema—loop diuretic prescribing cascade," *Journal of the American Pharmacists Association* 58, no. 5 (September-October 2018): 534-9. doi: 10.1016/j.japh.2018.06.014.

122 E. A. Davies and M. S. O'Mahony, "Adverse drug reactions in special populations—the elderly," *British Journal of Clinical Pharmacology* 80, no. 4 (October 2015): 796-807. doi: 10.1111/bcp.12596.

123 Robert L. Maher, Joseph Hanlon, and Emily R. Hajjar, "Clinical consequences of polypharmacy in elderly," *Expert Opinion on Drug Safety* 13, no. 1 (January 2014): 57-65. doi: 10.1517/14740338.2013.827660.

124 Bhavik M. Shah and Emily R. Hajjar, "Polypharmacy, adverse drug reactions, and geriatric syndromes," *Clinics in Geriatric Medicine* 28, no. 2 (May 2012): 173-186. doi: 10.1016/j.cger.2012.01.002.

125 Garber, "Medication overload: America's other drug problem."

126 Mark J. Rawle, Rachel Cooper, Diana Kuh, and Marcus Richards, "Associations between polypharmacy and cognitive and physical capability: a British cohort study," *Journal of the American Geriatric Society* 66, no. 5 (May 2018): 916-923.

127 Jonas W. Wastesson, Lucas Morin, Edwin C.K. Tan, and Kristina Johnell, "An update on the clinical consequences of polypharmacy in older adults, a narrative review," *Expert Opinion on Drug Safety* 17, no. 12 (2018): 1185-96.

128 Garber, "Medication overload: America's other drug problem."

129 Andrea Katsimpris, Jacob Linseisen, Christa Meisinger, and Konstantinos Volaklis, "The association between polypharmacy and physical function in older adults: a systematic review," *Journal of General Internal Medicine* 34, no. 9 (September 2019): 1865-73.

130 Claudine George amd Joe Verghese, "Polypharmacy and gait performance in community-dwelling older adults," *Journal of the American Geriatrics Society* 65, no. 9 (September 2017): 2082-2087. doi: 10.1111/jgs.14957.

131 Ibid.

132 Charlotte U. Andersen, Pernille O. Lassen, Hussain Q. Usman, Nadja Albertsen, Lars P. Nielsen, and Stig Andersen, "Prevalence of medication-related falls in 200

consecutive elderly patients with hip fractures: a cross-sectional study," *BMC Geriatrics* 20, no. 1 (March 30, 2020): 121. doi: 10.1186/s12877-020-01532-9.

133 Wastesson et al., "An update on the clinical consequences of polypharmacy in older adults, a narrative review."

134 Garber, "Medication overload: America's other drug problem."

135 Alonso Montiel-Luque, Antonio J. Nunez-Montenegro, Esther Martin-Aurioles, Jose C. Canca-Sanchez, Maria C. Toro-Toro, José A. Gonzalez-Correa, and Polipresact Research Group, "Medication-related factors associated with health-related quality of life in patient older than 65 years with polypharmacy," *PLoS One* 12, no. 2 (February 6, 2017): e0171320. doi: 10.1371/journal.pone.0171320.

136 Garber, et al., "Medication overload: America's other drug problem."

137 Working Group on Medication Overload, "Eliminating medication overload: a national action plan," Brookline, MA: The Lown Institute (2020).

138 Amy M. Linsky, Nancy R. Kressin, Kelly Stolzmann, Jacquelyn Pendergast, Amy K. Rosen, Barbara G. Bokhour, Steven R. Simon, "Direct-to-consumer strategies to promote deprescribing in primary care: a pilot study," *BMC Primary Care* 23, no. 1 (March 22, 2022): 53. doi: 10.1186/s12875-022-01655-5.

Chapter 6

139 Yoshita Paliwal, Resa M. Jones, Leticia R. Moczygemba, Tracey L. Gendron, Pramit A. Nadpara, Purva Parab, and Patricia W. Slattum, "Over-the-counter medication use in residents of senior living communities: a survey study," *Journal of the American Pharmacists Association* 61, no.6 (November-December 2021): 736-744. doi: 10.1016/j.japh.2021.05.023.

140 Richard R. Holden, Preethi Srinivas, Noll L. Campbell, Daniel O. Clark, Kunal S. Bodke, Youngbok Hong, Malaz A. Boustani, Denisha Ferguson, and Christopher M.Callahan, "Understanding older adults' medication decision making and behavior: a study on over-the-counter (OTC) anticholinergic medications" *Research in Social and Administrative Pharmacy* 15, no.1 (January 2019): 53-60. doi: 10.1016/j.sapharm.2018.03.002.

141 National Council on Patient Information and Education (now NeedyMeds at BeMedWise), "Empowering Americans to take greater responsibility for their health," 2020, (Accessed May 22, 2022), https://www.bemedwise.org /self-care-report/.

142 Janelle L. Sobotka and Barbara A. Kochanowski, "Self-Care and Nonprescription Pharmacotherapy," in Daniel L. Krinsky (Ed), *Handbook of nonprescription drugs, an interactive approach to self-care* (20th ed.), (Washington DC: American Pharmacists Association).

143   Drug Applications for Over-the-Counter (OTC) Drugs, March 31, 2020, US Food and Drug Administration, (Accessed June 8, 2022), https://www.fda.gov /drugs/types-applications/drug-applications-over-counter-otc-drugs.

144   Chelsey M. McIntyre and Gregory A. Heindel, "Dietary supplements: quality concerns and hospital formulary management," *P & T* 44, no.12 (201): 726-728, 730-731.

145   Elizabeth D. Kantor, Colin D. Rehm, Mengmeng Du, Emily White, and Edward L. Giovannucci, "Trends in dietary supplement use among US adults from 1999-2012," *Journal of the American Medical Association* 316, no.14 (October 11, 2016): 1464-74. doi: 10.1001/jama.2016.14403.

146   Dima M. Qato, Jocelyn Wilder, L. Philip Schumm, Victoria Gillet, and G. Caleb Alexander, "Changes in prescription and over-the-counter medication and dietary supplement use among older adults in the United States, 2005 vs 2011," *JAMA Intern Med* 176, no. 4 (2016): 473-82. doi: 10.1001/jamainternmed.2015.8581.

147   Suruchi Mishra, Bryan Stierman, Jaime J. Gahche, and Nancy Potischman, "Dietary supplement use among adults: United States, 2017-2018," *NCHS Data Brief* 399 (February 2021): 1-8.

148   Emily K. Farina, Krista G. Austin, and Harris R. Lieberman, "Concomitant dietary supplement and prescription medication use is prevalent among US adults with doctor-informed medical conditions," *Journal of the Academy of Nutrition and Dietetics* 114, no.11 (November 2014): 1784-90. doi: 10.1016/j.jand.2014.01.016.

149   Qato et al., "Changes in prescription and over-the-counter medication and dietary supplement use among older adults in the United States, 2005 vs 2011."

150   Drugs@FDA Glossary of Terms, Updated November 14, 2017, (Accessed May 24, 2022), https://www.fda.gov/drugs/drug-approvals-and-databases/drugsfda -glossary-terms#:~:text=or%20an%20injectable.-,Drug,any%20function%20 of%20the%20body.

151   US Food and Drug Administration, "Milestones of Drug Regulation in the United States," https://www.fda.gov/media/109482/download (Accessed September 1, 2022).

152   Ibid.

153   Over-the-counter (OTC) Drug Monograph Process, September 3, 2020, US Food and Drug Administration, (Accessed June 6, 2022), https://www.fda.gov /drugs/over-counter-otc-drug-monograph-process#:~:text=In%201972%2C%20 FDA%20established%20the,groups%20products%20by%20therapeutic%20 category.

154   Sobotka, *Handbook of nonprescription drugs, an interactive approach to self-care.*

155   Over-the-counter (OTC) Drug Monograph Process, September 3, 2020, US Food and Drug Administration, (Accessed June 6, 2022), https://www.fda.gov /drugs/over-counter-otc-drug-monograph-process#:~:text=In%201972%2C%20

FDA%20established%20the,groups%20products%20by%20therapeutic%20category.

156 Dietary Supplement Labeling Guide: Chapter 1, General Dietary Supplement Labeling, April 1, 2005, US Food and Drug Administration, (Accessed May 22, 2022), https://www.fda.gov/Food/GuidanceRegulation/GuidanceDocumentsRegulatoryInformation/DietarySupplements/ucm070519.htm.

157 Structure/function Claims, March 7, 2022, US Food and Drug Administration, (Accessed June 8, 2022), https://www.fda.gov/food/food-labeling-nutrition/structurefunction-claims.

158 McIntyre, et al., "Dietary supplements: quality concerns and hospital formulary management."

159 Guidance for industry: questions and answers regarding adverse event reporting and recordkeeping for dietary supplements as required by the dietary supplement and nonprescription drug consumer protection act, September 2013, US Food and Drug Administration (updated September 20, 2018), (Accessed June 8, 2022), https://www.fda.gov/regulatory-information/search-fda-guidance-documents/guidance-industry-questions-and-answers-regarding-adverse-event-reporting-and-recordkeeping-dietary#qa.

160 Randy C. Hatton and Leslie Hendeles, "Why is oral phenylephrine on the market after compelling evidence of its ineffectiveness as a decongestant?" *Annals of Pharmacotherapy* (published online March 25, 2022): https://doi.org/10.1177/10600280221081526.

161 Miles Weinberger and Leslie Hendeles, "Nonprescription medications for respiratory symptoms: facts and marketing fictions," *Allergy and Asthma Proceedings* 39, no. 3 (May-June 2018): 169-176.

162 Lombardi M, Carbone S, Giuseppe Del Buono M, et al., "Omega-3 fatty acids supplementation and risk of atrial fibrillation: an updated meta-analysis of randomized controlled trials (letter)," *European Heart Journal. Cardiovascular Pharmacotherapy* 7 no.4 (July 23, 2021): e69-e70. doi: 10.1093/ehjcvp/pvab008.

163 Stephanie Charles, Nidhi Agrawal, and Manfred Blum, "Erroneous thyroid diagnosis due to over-the-counter biotin," *Nutrition* 57 (January 2019): 257-258. Doi: 10.1016/j.nut.2018.05.005.

164 FDA in Brief: FDA reminds patients, health care professionals and laboratory personnel about the potential for biotin interference with certain test results, especially specific tests to aid in heart attack diagnoses, November 5, 2019, US Food and Drug Administration, (Accessed September 1, 2022), https://www.fda.gov/news-events/fda-brief/fda-brief-fda-reminds-patients-health-care-professionals-and-laboratory-personnel-about-potential.

165 Thomas J. Smith and Bimal H. Ashar, "Iron Deficiency Anemia Due to High-dose Turmeric," *Cureus* 11, no.1 (January 9, 2019): e3858. doi:10.7759/cureus.3858.

166 Andrew I. Geller, Nadine Shehab, Nina J. Weidle, Maribeth C. Lovegrove, Beverly J. Wolpert, Babgaleh B. Timbo, Robert P. Mozersky, and Daniel S. Budnitz, "Emergency department visits for adverse events related to dietary supplements," *New England Journal of Medicine* 373, no. 16 (October 15, 2015): 1531-1540. Doi: 10.1056/NEJMsa1504267.

167 Ibid.

168 McIntyre, et al., "Dietary supplements: quality concerns and hospital formulary management."

169 Michael C. White, "Dietary supplements pose real dangers to patients," *Annals of Pharmacotherapy* 54, no.8 (August 2020): 815-819. Doi: 10.1177/1060028019900504.

170 Archana Raghaven, Yoshita Paliwal, and Patricia W. Slattum. "Gaps in OTC labeling: potentially inappropriate medications for older adults," *The Consultant Pharmacist* 33, no. 3 (March 2018): 159-162.

171 Ibid.

172 Common medicines containing acetaminophen, (n.d.) (Accessed May 22, 2022), https://www.knowyourdose.org/common-medicines/.

173 Nichole L. Hodges, Henry A. Spiller, Marcel J. Casavant, Thiphalak Chounthirath, and Gary A. Smith, "Non-health care facility medication errors resulting in serious medical outcomes," *Clinical Toxicology* 56, no. 1 (January 2018): 43-50.

174 Clinical Resources, OTC brand-name extensions, (July 2021), Pharmacist's Letter/Prescriber's Letter [370709].

Chapter 7

175 Amanda D. Hutchinson, Dimitrios Saredakis, Rochelle Whelan, and Hannah A. Keage "Depression and its treatment in late life," *Senior Care Pharmacist* 35, no.12 (December 2020): 543-548. doi: 10.4140/TCP.n.2020.543.

176 Older Persons' Health, Leading Causes of Death, National Center for Health Statistics, (Accessed September 1, 2022), https://www.cdc.gov/nchs/fastats/older-american-health.htm.

177 Older Persons' Health, Obesity, National Center for Health Statistics, (Accessed September 1, 2022), https://www.cdc.gov/nchs/fastats/older-american-health.htm.

178 Centers for Disease Control and Prevention, "National Diabetes Statistics Report, 2020," Atlanta, GA: Centers for Disease Control and Prevention, U.S. Dept of Health and Human Services; 2020, (Accessed September 1, 2022), https://www.cdc.gov/diabetes/pdfs/data/statistics/national-diabetes-statistics-report.pdf.

179 American Diabetes Association Professional Practice Committee, "3. Prevention or delay of type 2 diabetes and associated comorbidities: Standards of Medical Care in Diabetes—2022," *Diabetes Care* 45, Suppl. 1 (January 2022): S39–S45. doi: 10.2337/dc22-S003.

180 *Geriatrics at your Fingertips*, 22nd edition, ed. David B. Reuben, Keela A. Herr, James T. Pacala, Bruce G. Pollock, Jane F. Potter, and Todd P. Semla (New York: American Geriatrics Society, 2020).

181 Chenchen Wang, Christopher H. Schmid, Maura D. Iversen, William F. Harvey, Roger A. Fielding, Jeffrey B. Driban, Lori Lyn Price, John B. Wong, Kieran F. Reid, Ramel Rones, and Timothy McAlindon, "Comparative Effectiveness of Tai Chi Versus Physical Therapy for Knee Osteoarthritis," *Annals of Internal Medicine* 165, no. 2 (July 19, 2016): 77-86. doi:10.7326/M15-2143.

182 Juyoung Park and Anne K. Hughes, "Nonpharmacological approaches to the management of chronic pain in community-dwelling older adults: a review of empirical evidence," *Journal of the American Geriatrics Society* 60, no.3 (March 2012): 555-568. doi: 10.1111/j.1532-5415.2011.03846.x.

183 Wang, et al., "Comparative Effectiveness of Tai Chi Versus Physical Therapy for Knee Osteoarthritis."

184 David Grimes, Megan Fitzpatrick, Joyce Gordon, Janis Miyasaki, Edward A. Fon, Michael Schlossmacher, et al., "Canadian guideline for Parkinson Disease," *Canadian Medical Association Journal* 191, no. 36 (September 9, 2019): E989-1004. doi: 10.1503/cmaj.181504.

185 Colin Binns, Peter Howat, James Smith, and Jonine Jancey, "The medicalisation of prevention: health promotion is more than a pill a day," (editorial) *Health Promotion Journal of Australia* 27, no.2 (August 2, 2016): 91-93. doi: 10.1071/HEv27n2_ED.

186 Donald M. Lloyd-Jones, Norrina B. Allen, Cheryl A.M. Anderson, Terrie Black, LaPrincess C. Brewer, Randi E. Forake, Michael A. Grandner, Helen Lavretsky, Amanda M. Perak, Garima Sharma, Wayne Rosamond, and American Heart Association, "Life's Essential 8: Updating and Enhancing the American Heart Association's Construct of Cardiovascular Health: A Presidential Advisory From the American Heart Association," *Circulation* 146, no.5 (August 2, 2022): e18-e43. doi: 10.1161/CIR.0000000000001078.

187 Anthony Komaroff, "Does sleep flush wastes from the brain?" (viewpoint) *Journal of the American Medical Association* 325, no. 21 (June 1, 2021): 2153-4. doi: 10.1001/jama.2021.5631.

188 Stephani Schrempft, Marta Jackowska, Mark Hamer, and Andrew Steptoe, "Associations between social isolation, loneliness, and objective physical activity in older men and women," *BMC Public Health* 19, no.1 (January 16, 2019): 74. doi: 10.1186/s12889-019-6424-y.

189 Thijs M.H. Eijsvogels and Paul D. Thompson, "Exercise is medicine, at any dose?" (viewpoint) *Journal of the American Medical Association* 314, no.18 (November 10, 2015): 1915-6. doi: 10.1001/jama.2015.10858.

190   Anon, "Fewer opioids, more exercise for severe joint pain from arthritis," *Journal of the American Medical Association* 316, no. 20 (November 22/29, 2016): 2079.

191   Shanhu Qiu, Xue Cai, Uwe Schumann, Martina Velders, Zilin Sun, and Jurgen M. Steinacker, "Impact of walking on glycemic control and other cardiovascular risk factors in type 2 diabetes: a meta-analysis," *PloSOne* 9, no.10 (October 17, 2014): e109767. doi: 10.1371/journal.pone.0109767.

192   Elaine M. Murtagh, Linda Nichols, Mohammed A. Mohammed, Roger Holder, Alan M. Nevill, and Marie H. Murphy, "The effect of walking on risk factors for cardiovascular disease: an updated systematic review and meta-analysis of randomised control trials," *Preventive Medicine* 72 (March 2015): 34-43. doi: 10.1016/j.ypmed.2014.12.041.

193   Klodian Dhana, Oscar H. Franco, Ethan M. Ritz, Christopher N. Ford, Pankaja Desai, Kristin R. Krueger, Thomas M. Holland, Anisa Dhana, Xiaoran Liu, Neelum t. Aggarwal, Denis a. Evans, and Kumar B. Rajan, "Healthy lifestyle and life expectancy with and without Alzheimer's dementia: population based cohort study," *British Medical Journal* 277 (April 13, 2022): e068390. doi: 10.1136/bmj-2021-068390.

194   Neil A. Kelly, Orysya Soroka, Chukwuma Onyebeke, Laura c. Pinheiro, Samprit Banerjee, Monika M. Saffort, and Parag Goyal, "Association of healthy lifestyle and all-cause mortality according to medication burden," *Journal of the American Geriatrics Society* 70 no. 2 (February 2022). doi: 10.1111/jgs.17521.

195   Gang Liu, Yanping Li, Yang Hu, Geng Zong, Shanshan Li, Eric B. Rimm, Frank B. Hu, JoAnn E. Manson, Kathryn M. Rexrode, Hyun J. Shin, and Qi Sun, "Influence of lifestyle on incident cardiovascular disease and mortality in patients with diabetes mellitus," *Journal of the American College of Cardiology* 71, no.25 (June 26, 2018): 2867-2876. doi: 10.1016/j.jacc.2018.04.027.

196   Kristin Franzon, Liisa Byberg, Per Sjögren, Björn Zethelius, Tommy Cederholm, and Lena Kilander, "Predictors of independent aging and survival: a 16-year follow-up report in octogenarian men," *Journal of the American Geriatrics Society* 65, no.9 (September 2017): 1953-1960. doi:10.1111/jgs.14971.

197   Liu et al., "Influence of lifestyle on incident cardiovascular disease and mortality in patients with diabetes mellitus."

198   Kelly et al., "Association of healthy lifestyle and all-cause mortality according to medication burden."

199   Ibid.

200   Franzon, et al., "Predictors of independent aging and survival: a 16-year follow-up report in octogenarian men."

201   Michael M. Pahor, Jack M. Guralnik, Walter T. Ambrosius, Steven Blair, Denise E. Bonds, Timothy S. Church, Mark A. Espeland, Roger A. Fielding, Thomas M. Gill, Erik J. Groessl, et al., "Effect of structured physical activity on prevention of

major mobility disability in older adults, the LIFE study randomized clinical trial," *Journal of the American Medical Association* 311, no. 23 (June 18, 2014): 2387-2396. doi: 10.1001/jama.2014.5616.

202 Liu et al., "Influence of lifestyle on incident cardiovascular disease and mortality in patients with diabetes mellitus."

203 Ute Mons, Aysel Müezzinler, Carolin Gellert, Ben Schöttker, Christian C. Abnet, Martin Bobak, Lisette de Groot, Neal D. Freedman, Eugène Jansen, Frank Kee, Daan Kromhout, Kari Kuulasmaa, et al., "Impact of smoking and smoking cessation on cardiovascular events and mortality among older adults: meta-analysis of individual participant data from prospective cohort studies of the CHANCES consortium," *British Medical Journal* 350 (April 20, 2015): h1551. doi: 10.1136/bmj.h1551.

204 Your Medicare Coverage, Medicare.gov, (accessed September 5, 2022), https://www.medicare.gov/coverage.

205 Stephen Devries, Walter Willett, and Robert O. Bonow, "Nutrition education in medical school, residency training, and practice" (viewpoint), *Journal of the American Medical Association* 321, no.14 (April 9, 2019): 1351-2. doi: 10.1001/jama.2019.1581.

206 H Foley, A. Steel, H. Cramer, J Wardle, and J. Adams, "Disclosure of complementary medicine use to medical providers: a systematic review and meta-analysis," *Scientific Reports* 9, no.1 (February 2019): 1573. doi: 10.1038/s41598-018-38279-8.

207 Elisabeth M.H. Mathus-Vliegen on behalf of the Obesity Management Task Force of the European Association for the Study of Obesity, "Prevalence, pathophysiology, health consequences and treatment options of obesity in the elderly: a guideline," *Obesity Facts* 5, no.3 (2012): 460-483. doi: 10.1159/000341193.

Chapter 8

208 Eric J. MacLaughlin, Cynthia L. Raehl, Angela Treadway, Teresa L. Sterling, Dennis P. Zoller, and Chester A. Bond, "Assessing medication adherence in the elderly," *Drugs and Aging* 22, no.3 (2005): 231-255.

209 Ibid.

210 Ibid.

211 Zachary A. Marcum, Joseph T. Hanlon, and Michael d. Murray, "Improving Medication Adherence and Health Outcomes in Older Adults An Evidence-Based Review of Randomized Controlled Trials," *Drugs and Aging* 34, no.3 (2017): 191-201. doi:10.1007/s40266-016-0433-7.

212 Carlotta Franchi, Ilaria Ardoino, Monica Ludergnani, Gjiliola Cukay, Luca Merlino, and Alessandro Nobili, "Medication adherence in community-dwelling older

people exposed to chronic polypharmacy," *Journal of epidemiology and community health* 75, no.9 (September 2021): 854-859. doi:10.1136/jech-2020-214238.

213 Michael A. Fischer, Niteesh K. Choudhry, Gregory Brill, Jerry Avorn, Sebastian Schneeweiss, David Hutchins, Joshua N. Liberman, Toryen A. Brennan, and William H. Shrank, "Trouble getting started: predictors of primary medication nonadherence," *The American Journal of Medicine* 124, no. 11 (November 2011): 1081.e9-22. doi:10.1016/j.amjmed.2011.05.028.

214 Franchi, "Medication adherence in community-dwelling older people exposed to chronic polypharmacy."

215 Ibid.

216 Aurel O. Iuga and Maura J. McGuire, "Adherence and health care costs," *Risk Management and Healthcare Policy* 20, no. 7 (February 2014): 35-44. doi:10.2147/RMHP.S19801.

217 Caroline A. Walsh, Caitriona Cahir, and Kathleen E. Bennett, "Longitudinal medication adherence in older adults with multmorbidity and association with health care utilization: results from the Irish Longitudinal Study on Ageing," *Annals of Pharmacotherapy* 55, no.1 (2021): 5-14. doi: 10.1177/1060028020937996.

218 Iuga, "Adherence and health care costs."

219 Fred Kleinsinger, "The unmet challenge of medication nonadherence," *The Permanente Journal* 22 (2018): 18-033. doi: 10.7812/TPP/18-033.

220 Iuga, "Adherence and health care costs."

221 Joseph Bubalo, Roger K. Clark Jr., Susie S. Jiing, Nathan B. Johnson, Katherine A. Miller, Colleen J. Clemens-Shipman, and Amanda L. Sweet, "Medication adherence: pharmacists perspective," *Journal of the American Pharmacists Association* 50, no. 3 (May/June 2010): 394-406.

222 Maclaughlin, "Assessing medication adherence in the elderly."

223 Colleen A. McHorney and Abhijit S. Gadkari, "Individual patients hold different beliefs to prescription medications to which they persist vs nonpersist and persist vs nonfulfill," *Patient preference and adherence* 4 (2010): 187-95. doi:10.2147/ppa.s10603.

224 Franchi, "Medication adherence in community-dwelling older people exposed to chronic polypharmacy."

225 Kunal Srivastava, Anamika Arora, Aditi Kataria, Joseph C. Cappelleri, Alesia Sadosky, and Andrew M. Peterson, "Impact of reducing dosing frequency on adherence to oral therapies: a literature review and meta-analysis," *Patient preference and adherence* 7 (2013): 419-434.

226 Maclaughlin, "Assessing medication adherence in the elderly."

227 Megan N. Wilson, Christopher L. Greer, and Douglas L. Weeks, "Medication regimen complexity and hospital readmission for an adverse drug event," *Annals of Pharmacotherapy* 48, no. 1 (January 2014): 26-32. doi: 10.1177/1060028013510898.

228 Kirsi Kvarnström, Aleksi Westerholm, Marja Airaksinen, and Helena Liira, "Factors Contributing to Medication Adherence in Patients with a Chronic Condition: A Scoping Review of Qualitative Research," *Pharmaceutics* 13, no. 7 (July 2021): 1100. doi: 10.3390/pharmaceutics13071100.

229 David Yiu, Annie Lam, and Czarina Franco, "Assessing medication nonadherence among community dwelling older adults," *The Consultant Pharmacist* 29, no. 10 (October 2014): 676.

230 Eduardo Sabaté, *Adherence to long-term therapies: evidence for action*, (Geneva: World Health Organization, 2003).

231 Yiu, "Assessing medication nonadherence among community dwelling older adults."

232 Kvarnström, "Factors Contributing to Medication Adherence in Patients with a Chronic Condition: A Scoping Review of Qualitative Research."

233 Hedva B. Levy and Karen Frank Barney, "Pharmacology, pharmacy, and the aging adults: implications for occupational therapy," in *Occupational Therapy with Aging Adults*, 2nd ed. Karen Frank Barney and Margaret A. Perkinson (St. Louis: Elsevier, in press).

234 Sabaté, *Adherence to long-term therapies: evidence for action*.

235 McHorney, "Individual patients hold different beliefs to prescription medications to which they persist vs nonpersist and persist vs nonfulfill."

236 Ibid.

Chapter 9

237 By the 2023 American Geriatrics Society Beers Criteria® Update Expert Panel, "American Geriatrics Society 2023 Updated AGS Beers Criteria® for Potentially Inappropriate Medication Use in Older Adults," *Journal of the American Geriatrics Society* 71 (e-pub May 4, 2023): 1-30. doi: 10.1111/jgs.18372.

238 Lisa E. Hines and John E. Murphy, "Potentially harmful drug-drug interactions in the elderly: a review," *American Journal of Geriatric Pharmacotherapy* 9, no. 6 (December 2011): 367-77.

239 Louse Mallet, Anne Spinewine, and Allen Huang, "Prescribing in elderly people 2, the challenge of managing drug interactions in elderly people," *Lancet* 370, no. 9582 (2007): 185-91.

240 Archana Raghaven, Yoshita Paliwal, and Patricia W. Slattum, "Gaps in OTC labeling: potentially inappropriate medications for older adults," *Consultant Pharmacist* 33, no.3 (March 2018): 159-162.

241   Alison A. Moore, Elizabeth J. Whiteman, and Katherine T. Ward, "Risks of combined alcohol-medication use in older adults," *American Journal of Geriatric Pharmacotherapy* 5, no. 1 (March 2007): 64-74.

242   Joshua D. Brown and Almut G. Winterstein, "Potential adverse drug events and drug-drug interactioons with medical and consumer cannabidiol (CBD) use," *Journal of Clinical Medicine* 8, no.7 (July 2019): 989.

243   Bhavik Shah and Emily R. Hajjar, "Polypharmacy, adverse drug reactions, and geriatric syndromes," *Clinics in Geriatric Medicine* 28, no. 2 (May 2012): 173-186.

244   Louise Mallet, Anne Spinewine, and Allen Huang, "Prescribing in elderly people 2, the challenge of managing drug interactions in elderly people." *Lancet* 370, no. 9582 (July 14, 2007): 185-191.

245   Amanda Lavan and Paul Gallagher, "Predicting risk of adverse drug reactions in older adults," *Therapeutic Advances in Drug Safety* 7, no. 1 (2016): 11-22.

246   Jennifer Panich, Andrea Gooden, F. Mazda Shirazi, and Daniel C. Malone, "Warnings for drug-drug interactions in consumer medication information provided by community pharmacies," *Journal of the American Pharmacists Association* 59 (2019): 35-42.

Chapter 10

247   Collin M. Clark, Amy L. Shaver, Leslie A. Aurelio, Steven Feuerstein, Robert G. Wahler Jr., Christopher J. Daly, and David M. Jacobs, "Potentially inappropriate medications are associated with increased healthcare utilization and costs," *Journal of the American Geriatrics Society* 68, no.11 (November 2020): 2542-2550.

248   Ibid.

249   Agency for Healthcare Research and Quality, 2018 National Healthcare Quality and Disparities Report, Chartbook on Patient Safety AHRQ 2018.

250   Michael Fralick, Emily Bartsch, Christine S. Ritchie, and Chana A. Sacks, "Estimating the use of potentially inappropriate medications among older adults tin the United States," *Journal of the American Geriatrics Society* 68, no. 12 (December 2020): 2927-2930.

251   Mark H. Beers, Joseph G. Ouslander, Irving Rollingher, David B. Reuben, Jacqueline Brooks, and John C. Beck, "Explicit criteria for determining inappropriate medication use in nursing home residents," *Archives of Internal Medicine* 151, no.9 (September 1991): 1825-1832.

252   By the 2023 American Geriatrics Society Beers Criteria® Update Expert Panel, "American Geriatrics Society 2023 Updated AGS Beers Criteria® for Potentially Inappropriate Medication Use in Older Adults," *Journal of the American Geriatrics Society* 71 (e-pub May 4, 2023): 1-30. doi: 10.1111/jgs.18372.

253   Beers et al., "Explicit criteria for determining inappropriate medication use in nursing home residents."

254 By the 2023 American Geriatrics Society Beers Criteria® Update Expert Panel, "American Geriatrics Society 2023 Updated AGS Beers Criteria® for Potentially Inappropriate Medication Use in Older Adults."

255 Denis O'Mahony, David O'Sullivan, Stephen Byrne, Marie N. O'Connor, Cristin Ryan, and Paul Gallagher, "STOPP/START criteria for potentially inappropriate prescribing in older people: version 2," *Age and Ageing* 44, no. 2 (March 2015): 213-218. doi: 10.1093/ageing/afu145; Erratum in: *Age and Ageing* 47, no. 3 (May 2018): 489.

256 Marisa Bare, Marina Lleal, Sara Ortonobes, Maria Queralt Gogas, Daniel Sevilla-Sanchez, Nuria Carballo, et al., "Factors associated to potentially inappropriate prescribing in older patients according to STOPP/START criteria: MoPIM multicentre cohort study," *BMC Geriatrics* 22 (2022): 44. https://doi.org/10.1186/s12877-021-02715-8.

257 Martin Taylor-Rowan, Sophie Edwards, Anna H Noel-Storr, Jenny McCleery, Phyo K Myint, Roy Soiza, Carrie Stewart, Yoon K Loke, and Terry J Quinn, "Anticholinergic burden (prognostic factor) for prediction of dementia or cognitive decline in older adults with no known cognitive syndrome," *Cochrane Database of Systematic Reviews* (2021), Issue 5. Art. No.: CD013540. doi: 10.1002/14651858. CD013540.pub2.

258 Laura E. Targownik, Deborah A. Fisher, and Sameer D. Saini, "AGA clinical practice update on de-prescribing of proton pump inhibitors," *Gastroenterology* 162 (April 2022): 1334-42.

259 Katy E. Trinkley, Allison M. Sturm, Kyle Porter, and Milap C. Nahata, "Efficacy and Safety of Atypical Antipsychotics for Behavioral and Psychological Symptoms of Dementia Among Community Dwelling Adults," *Journal of Pharmacy Practice* 33, no.1 (January 2020): 7-14.

260 Annya Tisher and Arash Salardini, "A comprehensive update on treatment of dementia," *Seminars in Neurology* 39, no.2 (2019):167-178.doi:10.1055/s-0039-1683408.

261 American Geriatrics Society, "Tip Sheet: What To Do And What To Ask If A Medication You Take Is Listed In The AGS Beers Criteria® For Potentially Inappropriate Medication Use In Older Adults," https://www.healthinaging.org/tools-and-tips/tip-sheet-what-do-and-what-ask-if-medication-you-take-listed-ags`-beers-criteriar.

Chapter 11

262 By the 2023 American Geriatrics Society Beers Criteria® Update Expert Panel, "American Geriatrics Society 2023 Updated AGS Beers Criteria® for Potentially Inappropriate Medication Use in Older Adults," *Journal of the American Geriatrics Society* 71 (e-pub May 4, 2023): 1-30. doi: 10.1111/jgs.18372.

263 Nadine Shehab, Maribeth C. Lovegrove, Andrew I. Geller, Kathleen O. Rose, Nina J. Weidle, and Daniel S. Budnitz, "US Emergency Department Visits for

Outpatient Adverse Drug Events, 2013-2014," *Journal of the American Medical Association* 316, no. 20 (November 22/29, 2016): 2115-2125.

264 Daniel S. Budnitz, Nadine Shehab, Maribeth C. Lovegrove, Andrew J. Geller, Jennifer N. Lind, and Daniel A. Pollock, "US Emergency Department Visits Attributed to Medication Harms, 2017-2019," *Journal of the American Medical Association* 326, no. 13 (October 5, 2021): 1299-1309.

265 U.S. Department of Health and Human Services, Office of Disease Prevention and Health Promotion, "National Action Plan for Adverse Drug Event Prevention," (Washington, DC, 2014) PDF accessed online July 12, 2022: https://health.gov/our-work/national-health-initiatives/health-care-quality/adverse-drug-events/national-ade-action-plan.

266 Budnitz et al., "US Emergency Department Visits Attributed to Medication Harms, 2017-2019."

267 Ibid.

268 Badieh Jafari and Mary E. Britton, "Hypoglycaemia in elderly patients with type 2 diabetes mellitus: a review of risk factors, consequences and prevention," *Journal of Pharmacy Practice and Research* 45, no.4 (December 2015): 459–469. doi: 10.1002/jppr.1163.

269 Jennifer G. Naples, Walid F. Gellad, and Joseph T. Hanlon, "Managing pain in older adults: the role of opioid analgesics," *Clinics in Geriatric Medicine* 32, no.4 (November 2016): 725-735.

270 By the 2023 American Geriatrics Society Beers Criteria® Update Expert Panel, "American Geriatrics Society 2023 Updated AGS Beers Criteria® for Potentially Inappropriate Medication Use in Older Adults."

271 Shoshana J. Herzig, Timothy S. Anderson, Yoojin Jung, Long H. Ngo, and Ellen P. McCarthy, "Risk factors for opioid-related adverse drug events among older adults after hospital discharge," *Journal of the American Geriatrics Society* 70, no.1 (January 2022): 228-234.

272 By the 2023 American Geriatrics Society Beers Criteria® Update Expert Panel, "American Geriatrics Society 2023 Updated AGS Beers Criteria® for Potentially Inappropriate Medication Use in Older Adults."

273 Denis O'Mahony, David O'Sullivan, Stephen Byrne, Marie N. O'Connor, Cristin Ryan, and Paul Gallagher, "STOPP/START criteria for potentially inappropriate prescribing in older people: version 2," *Age and Ageing* 44, no.2 (March 2015): 213-218.

274 Martin Taylor-Rowan, Sophie Edwards, Anna H Noel-Storr, Jenny McCleery, Phyo K Myint, Roy Soiza Carrie Stewart, Yoon Kong Loke, and Terry J Quinn, "Anticholinergic burden (prognostic factor) for prediction of dementia or cognitive decline in older adults with no known cognitive syndrome," *Cochrane Database*

of Systematic Reviews, (2021) 5 Art. No.: CD013540. doi: 10.1002/14651858. CD013540.pub2.

275 Centers for Disease Control and Prevention, "Older adult fall prevention," September 6, 2022. (Accessed September 15, 2022), https://www.cdc.gov/falls/index.html.

276 By the 2023 American Geriatrics Society Beers Criteria® Update Expert Panel, "American Geriatrics Society 2023 Updated AGS Beers Criteria® for Potentially Inappropriate Medication Use in Older Adults."

277 O'Mahony et al., "STOPP/START criteria for potentially inappropriate prescribing in older people: version 2."

278 By the 2023 American Geriatrics Society Beers Criteria® Update Expert Panel, "American Geriatrics Society 2023 Updated AGS Beers Criteria® for Potentially Inappropriate Medication Use in Older Adults."

Chapter 12

279 Georgie B. Lee, Christopher Etherton-Beer, Sarah M. Hosking, Julie A. Pasco, and Amy T. Page, "The patterns and implications of potentially suboptimal medicine regimens among older adults: a narrative review," *Therapeutic advances in drug safety* 13 (July 4, 2022): 1-41. doi:10.1177/20420986221100117.

280 Maarten Wauters, Monique Elseviers, Bert Vaes, Jan Degryse, Olivia Dalleur, Robert Vander Stichele, Thierry Chistiaens, and Majda Azermai, "Too many, too few, or too unsafe? Impact of inappropriate prescribing on mortality, and hospitalization in a cohort of community-dwelling oldest old," *British Journal of Clinical Pharmacology* 82, no.5 (2016): 1382-1392. doi:10.1111/bcp.13055.

281 Ibid.

282 Roger E. Thomas, Leonard T. Nguyen, Dave Jackson, and Christopher Naugler, "Potentially Inappropriate Prescribing and Potential Prescribing Omissions in 82,935 Older Hospitalised Adults: Association with Hospital Readmission and Mortality within Six Months," *Geriatrics* (Basel, Switzerland) 5, no. 2 (June 12, 2020): 37. doi:10.3390/geriatrics5020037

283 Lee, et al., "The patterns and implications of potentially suboptimal medicine regimens among older adults: a narrative review."

284 Ibid.

285 Cynthia M. Boyd, Jonathan Darer, Chad Boult, Linda P. Fried, Lisa Boult, and Albert W. Wu, "Clinical practice guidelines and quality of care for older patients with multiple comorbid diseases," *Journal of the American Medical Association* 294, no. 6 (August 10, 2005): 716-24.

286 Denis O'Mahony, David O'Sullivan, Stephen Byrne, Marie N. O'Connor, Cristin Ryan, and Paul Gallagher, "STOPP/START criteria for potentially inappropriate prescribing in older people: version 2," *Age and Ageing* 44, no.2 (March 2015):

213-218. doi: 10.1093/ageing/afu145, Erratum in: *Age and Ageing* 47, no. 3 (May 2018): 489.

287 Antonio Cherubini, Andrea Corsonello, and Fabrizia Lattanzio, "Underprescription of beneficial medications in older people," *Drugs and Aging* 29, no. 6 (2012): 463-475.

288 Terri R. Fried and Marcia C. Mecca, "Medication appropriateness in vulnerable older adults: a healthy skepticism of appropriate polypharmacy," *Journal of the American Geriatrics Society* 67, no. 6 (June 2019): 1123-1127.

289 Karen L. Pellegrin, Elizabeth Lee, Reece Uyeno, Chris Ayson, and Roy Goo, "Potentially preventable medication-related hospitalizations: a clinical pharmacist approach to assessment, categorization, and quality improvement," *Journal of the American Pharmacists Association* 57 (2017): 711-716.

Chapter 13

290 J Garber and S Brownlee, *Medication Overload: America's Other Drug Problem*, (Brookline, MA: The Lown Institute, 2019), 4, https://lowninstitute.org/projects/medication-overload-how-the-drive-to-prescribe-is-harming-older-americans/.

291 Working Group on Medication Overload, "Eliminating medication overload: a national action plan," (Brookline, MA: The Lown Institute, 2020). https://lowninstitute.org/reports/eliminating-medication-overload-a-national-action-plan/.

292 Advocate, Merriam-Webster Dictionary, (accessed September 8, 2022), https://www.merriam-webster.com/dictionary/advocate.

293 The American Geriatrics Society Expert Panel on Person-centered Care, "Person-centered care: a definition and essential elements," *Journal of the American Geriatrics Society* 64, no. 1 (January 2016): 15-8.

Chapter 14

294 US Food and Drug Administration, Frequently asked questions on patents and exclusivity, February 5, 2020. https://www.fda.gov/drugs/development-approval-process-drugs/frequently-asked-questions-patents-and-exclusivity#What_is_the_difference_between_patents_a (Accessed September 1, 2022).

295 Denis O'Mahony, David O'Sullivan, Stephen Byrne, Marie N. O'Connor, Cristin Ryan, and Paul Gallagher, "STOPP/START criteria for potentially inappropriate prescribing in older people: version 2," *Age and Ageing* 44, no. 2 (March 2015): 213-218. doi: 10.1093/ageing/afu145. Erratum in: *Age and Ageing* 47, no. 3 (May 2018): 489.

296 Ibid.

297 Mayo Clinic, Dry mouth, https://www.mayoclinic.org/diseases-conditions/dry-mouth/symptoms-causes/syc-20356048, (Accessed September 1, 2022).

298 US Food and Drug Administration, "FDA drug safety communication: special storage and handling requirements must be followed for Pradaxa (dabigatran etexilate mesylate) capsules," (March 29, 2011), https://www.fda.gov/drugs /drug-safety-and-availability/fda-drug-safety-communication-special-storage-and -handling-requirements-must-be-followed-pradaxa, (Accessed August 1, 2022).

Chapter 15

299 O. Laatikainen, S. Sneck, and M. Turpeinen, "Medication-related adverse events in health care—what have we learned? A narrative overview of the current knowledge," *European Journal of Pharmacology* 78, no.2 (February 2022): 159-170. doi: 10.1007/s00228-021-03213-x.

300 Institute of Medicine (US) Committee on Quality of Health Care in America, *To Err is Human: Building a Safer Health System*, Edited by Linda T. Kohn, Janet M. Corrigan, and Molla S. Donaldson, (US: National Academies Press, 2000). doi:10.17226/9728.

301 Institute of Medicine, *Preventing Medication Errors*, (Washington, DC: The National Academies Press, 2007). https://doi.org/10.17226/11623.

302 Medication Errors: Technical Series on Safer Primary Care, (Geneva: World Health Organization, 2016). Licence: CC BY-NC-SA 3.0 IGO.

303 Ibid.

304 Institute of Medicine, *Preventing Medication Errors.*

305 Christopher M. Wittich, Christopher M. Burkle, and William L. Lanier, "Medication errors: an overview for clinicians," *Mayo Clinic Proceedings* 89, no. 8 (2014): 1116-1125.

306 Ibid.

307 World Health Organization, Medication Safety Without Harm, (Accessed September 1, 2022), https://www.who.int/initiatives/medication-without-harm.

308 Institute of Medicine. *Preventing Medication Errors.*

309 Jerry H. Gurwitz, Terry S. Field, Leslie R. Harrold, Jeffrey Rothschild, Kristin Debellis, Andrew C. Seger, Cynthia Cadoret, Leslie S. Fish, Lawrence Garber, Michael Kelleher, and David W. Bates, "Incidence and preventability of adverse drug events among older persons in the ambulatory setting," *Journal of the American Medical Association* 289, no. 9 (March 5, 2003): 1107-1116.

310 Terry S. Field, Boyd H. Gilman, Sujha Subramanian, Jackie C. Fuller, David W. Bates, and Jerry H. Gurwitz, "The costs associated with adverse drug events among older adults in the ambulatory setting," *Medical Care* 43, no. 12 (December 2005): 1171-1176.

311　Nichole L. Hodges, Henry A. Spiller, Marcel J. Casavant, Thiphalak Chounthirath, and Gary A. Smith, "Non-health care facility medication errors resulting in serious medical outcomes," *Clinical Toxicology* 56, no. 1 (2018): 43-50.

312　Ibid.

313　Gurwitz et al., "Incidence and preventability of adverse drug events among older persons in the ambulatory setting."

314　Ibid.

315　Terry S. Field, Kathleen M. Mazor, Becky Briesacher, Kristin R. Debellis, and Jerry H. Gurwitz, "Adverse drug events resulting from patient errors in older adults," *Journal of the American Geriatrics Society* 55, no. 2 (February 2007): 271-276. doi:10.1111/j.1532-5415.2007.01047.x.

316　Assiri, et al., "What is the epidemiology of medication errors, error-related adverse events and risk factors for errors in adults managed in community care contexts? A systematic review of the international literature."

317　Medication Errors: Technical Series on Safer Primary Care, p 19.

318　Institute of Safe Medication Practices, "Key elements of medication use," (accessed August 31, 2022), https://www.ismp.org/key-elements-medication-use.

Chapter 16

319　American Diabetes Association Professional Practice Committee, "Older adults, standards of care in diabetes 2022," *Diabetes Care* 45, suppl. 11 (January 2022): S195–S207. https://doi.org/10.2337/dc22-S013.

320　Amir Qaseem, Devan Kansagara, Mary Ann Forciea, Molly Cooke, and Thomas D. Denberg, "Management of chronic insomnia disorder in adults: a clinical practice guideline from the American College of Physicians," *Annals Internal Medicine* 165, no. 2 (July 19, 2016): 125-133.

321　Barbara Farrell, Emily Galley, Lianne Jeffs, Pam Howell, and Lisa M. McCarthy, "'Kind of blurry': Deciphering clues to prevent, investigate and manage prescribing cascades, *PLOS One* 17, no. 8 (August 31, 2022): e0272418.

322　By the 2023 American Geriatrics Society Beers Criteria® Update Expert Panel, "American Geriatrics Society 2023 Updated AGS Beers Criteria® for Potentially Inappropriate Medication Use in Older Adults," *Journal of the American Geriatrics Society* 71 (e-pub May 4, 2023): 1-30. doi: 10.1111/jgs.18372.

323　Choosing Wisely, "Our Mission," (accessed September 1, 2022), https://www.choosingwisely.org/our-mission/.

Chapter 17

324　Imran Ahmed, Niall S. Ahmad, Shahnaz Ali, Shari Ali, Anju George, Hiba Saleem Danish, Encarl Uppal, James Soo, Mohammad H. Mobasheri, Dominic King,

Benita Cox, and Ara Darzi, "Medication Adherence Apps: Review and Content Analysis," *JMIR Mhealth and Uhealth* 6, no. 3 (March 2018): e62, https://mhealth.jmir.org/2018/3/e62. doi: 10.2196/mhealth.6432.

325 Claudine Backes, Carla Moyano, Camille Rimaud, Christine Bienvenu, and Marie P. Schneider, "Digital Medication Adherence Support: Could Healthcare Providers Recommend Mobile Health Apps?" *Frontiers in Medical Technology* 2 (February 17, 2021): 616242, https://www.frontiersin.org/articles/10.3389/fmedt.2020.616242. doi: 10.3389/fmedt.2020.616242.

326 Ibid.

327 Sadaf Faisal, Jessica Ivo, and Tejal Patel, "A review of features and characteristics of smart medication adherence products," *Canadian Pharmacists Journal* 154, no.5 (September/October 2021): 312-323. doi: 10.1177/17151635211034198.

Chapter 18

328 By the 2023 American Geriatrics Society Beers Criteria® Update Expert Panel, "American Geriatrics Society 2023 Updated AGS Beers Criteria® for Potentially Inappropriate Medication Use in Older Adults," *Journal of the American Geriatrics Society* 71 (e-pub May 4, 2023): 1-30. doi: 10.1111/jgs.18372.

329 Joshua Davis Kinsey and Diane Nykamp, "Dangers of nonprescription medicines: educating and counseling older adults," *The Consultant Pharmacist* 32, no. 5 (May 2017): 269-280.

330 Michael C. White, "Dietary supplements pose real dangers to patients," *Annals of Pharmacotherapy* 54, no.8 (August 2020) :815-819. doi: 10.1177/1060028019900504.

Index

NOTES

NOTES

NOTES

NOTES

NOTES

NOTES

NOTES

NOTES

NOTES

NOTES

NOTES

NOTES

NOTES

NOTES

NOTES

NOTES

NOTES